NEW CONCEPTS IN BLOOD FORMATION AND CELL GENERATION
in Malignant and Benign Tissues

Volume II

Cardiac Muscle

Adult and embryonic tissues from humans and animals;
and in chronic ischemic conditions, acute rheumatic fever,
and coronary occlusion with myocardial infarction.

HEMPROVA GHOSH McDONALD, M.D., F.C.A.P.
Director, Diagnostic and Cell Research Institute
Waco, Texas

DIAGNOSTIC AND CELL RESEARCH INSTITUTE
WACO, TEXAS
1995

Published by:
Diagnostic and Cell Research Institute
P. O. Box 7216
Waco, Texas 76710-7216

Library of Congress Catalog Number: 89-90849

ISBN Number: 0-9627824-1-6

PRINTED IN THE UNITED STATES OF AMERICA
BY DAVIS PUBLISHING COMPANY, WACO, TEXAS

DEDICATION

This book and those to come in the future
are dedicated to the Almighty God, who has
given power to my eyes to see, the ability of
my mind to analyze, and has provided in me
a great desire and perseverance to continue
these basic cellular studies year after year.

Preface and Acknowledgements: Volume II

My research in cell life began in 1951 when I was awarded a fellowship in cancer research at the Washington University School of Medicine, St. Louis, Missouri. I began by focusing on cellular changes in epidermis in development of squamous cell carcinoma in an experimental carcinogenesis project. As my research progressed over the years, I began to notice that cells were arising without undergoing mitosis. (Mitosis is found to be rather rare for generation of cells particularly in benign tissues.) At first, I myself did not want to believe that this was possible, but as I accumulated more and more information through the critical study of thousands of tissue sections, it became undeniable.

Further investigation revealed that many types of processes were involved in nonmitotic cell generation. Some of these processes were demonstrated with photomicrographs in several scientific publications and also presented at the annual meetings of several professional organizations between 1957 and 1986.

New Concepts in Blood Formation and Cell Generation in Malignant and Benign Tissues, Volume I, was published in 1989. Although I had originally intended to publish only one book, the enormous diversity of information compelled me to divide the material into groups. The first volume concentrated on the essential developmental processes seen in and near cancer, while only briefly demonstrating the similarities seen in benign tissues. In that volume the 'new concepts' in mechanisms of origin, growth, metastasis, and local invasion are briefly pointed out with photomicrographs in a few tumors. The transformation processes of cancerous tissues into benign forms (including fibrous stroma, blood, blood vessels, and reactive or inflammatory cells) are demonstrated in breast carcinomas, skin cancers, and carcinomas of colon, kidney and prostate. It is hoped that in future volumes based on my experience more discussions will be presented regarding the life cycles of various additional benign and malignant tissues.

Because of the many important observations that I have made in cardiac muscle, which I would like to share with the readers, I decided to devote this second volume entirely to cardiac muscle (both apparently normal muscle and muscle involved in a few well-known cardiac ailments). Most of the structural changes that I have observed and studied in cardiac muscle are included in this volume.

A long-awaited discussion of the diverse ways of blood formation (red cells, white blood cells, and platelets) in bone marrow of apparently normal individuals as well as individuals suffering from some hematological disorders will be presented in yet another volume.

Throughout my investigative career, spanning over four decades, many people assisted me immensely in different ways. I gratefully acknowledged my indebtedness to those persons in my first volume in 1989. I am greatly indebted to Dr. Wilbur A. Thomas, then a Senior faculty member in the General Pathology Department of Washington University School of Medicine, for allowing me access to autopsy material of patients who died of acute rheumatic fever mostly before the advent of antibiotics.

My thankfulness to Rani Ghosh, Dan Browder, Jeff DeLoach, Julie Rothe, Jo Ann Lee, Amanda Heidemann, and Bernard Machovsky for their help in the preparation of this manuscript. Bernard Machovsky and Rani Ghosh proved to be invaluable in their assistance in publication of this book.

Finally, I wish again, to express my heartfelt thanks and great appreciation to my husband, Dr. Hendley A. McDonald, who has continued to be my source of encouragement and has contributed many valuable suggestions in preparation of the manuscript.

I greatly appreciate the permission for reproduction of my three articles on Acute Rheumatic Fever given by the editors and publishers of the following journals: *Texas State Journal of Medicine, Journal of Clinical Pathology*, and *Experimental Pathology*. These articles are reproduced in the Appendix (pages 88-117).

Waco, Texas
1995

Hemprova G. McDonald, M. D.

Preface and Acknowledgements: Volume I

Author's Note: The Preface and Acknowledgements of Volume I are reprinted here to acknowledge the many individuals and organizations who have contributed to the author's past and present research efforts.

As I ventured to write a book on my microscopic findings with the experience of thirty years of study of human and animal tissues, I thought that in the preface I should express my habit of viewing morphological structures as a phase of continuous transformation. I also inquire into their possible past and future developmental processes, which have helped me to unveil many actual and logical sequences of events leading to the solution of some biological problems. The presence of blood outside vascular channels need not be interpreted as hemorrhage simply because of the preconceived idea that blood cannot be formed other than in bone marrow and only through nucleated phases of erythropoiesis. In fact, this book and future volumes will show the possibilities of different ways of red cell formation directly as hemoglobin globules from practically every organ and tissue of the body, including bone marrow.

I am indebted to many persons from my college years until present times who have encouraged and are still encouraging me and helping in my investigative work involving cells and tissues. I am even indebted to those reviewers who repeatedly discouraged me by not accepting my manuscripts for publication in their journals, usually with the remark that it would be better suited for other types of journals. These refusals no doubt dampened my spirit initially, but resulted in a deeper and expanded study of my field of investigation as I prepared yet another paper just to be refused again.

I understand that it is not easy to spread views which oppose the generally accepted theories on histogenesis of various morphological structures, even though in no available literature does one find a demonstration of the accepted views as clear as that which I present here. I have been repeatedly advised by professional well-wishers that I should work in the line of generally accepted belief, and would as a result encounter fewer problems in publication. That was certainly true, since I had encountered no problems in my earlier publications of a clinical nature which evoked no controversy. Many years passed during which I have accumulated a vast amount of unpublished data based on my original work, of which only a small portion has been published. Now, avoiding more unnecessary delay, I am determined to publish, on my own, my findings in a series of books dealing with cell generation, differentiation and transformation covering various tissues, ma-lignant and benign, both in humans and animals (mainly in mice). The first volume concerns neoplasms and a few illustrations from benign tissues including bone marrow. Various benign tissues and additional neoplastic tissues will be included in later volumes.

I believe that the demonstrations in this book dealing with various pathways of cell generation and transformation in development of different morphological structures can easily be followed by an unbiased mind, and, hopefully, would create more interest in observation and analysis of the life cycles of various cells and tissues.

My investigative career started while I was a medical student at Calcutta Medical College (Calcutta University, India). After graduation I devoted my time both to clinical medicine and experimental work in immunology. I was stimulated in creating a mind for research by my cousin, a renowned scientist, the late Dr. B. C. Guha, chairman of the Department of Biochemistry, Calcutta University, and by the late Dr. J. C. Ray, director and founder of the Indian Institute for Medical Research, Calcutta. A long association with Dr. Ray and also with Dr. A.N. Roy of the same institute furthered my research career.

It was not until 1951 that I began my investigative work on cell life when I was awarded a Danforth Foundation Fellowship by the Washington University School of Medicine, St. Louis, Missouri, with the recommendation of Dr. E. V. Cowdry, the head of the Cancer Research Division, and his friend from India, Dr. S.C. Ray.

While I was carrying out cytological studies of experimental chemical carcinogenesis using epidermis of mice, I became aware that in order to enlarge my field of study I needed to gain more knowledge in the area of pathology of tumors. With that ambition, after finishing my general pathology training at St. Louis City Hospital, I took surgical pathology training at Washington University under Dr. Lauren V. Ackerman. After the completion of training, I held the position of Instructor of Surgical Pathology at the same institution until 1959. During my association with the surgical pathology division I was carrying out a small scale experimental cancer chemotherapy program, using mainly mammary carcinomas in mice. This program was sponsored by the Glover H. Copher Fund at Washington University.

Because of the critical microscopic examination of mammary tumors and benign tissues of experimental and control groups of mice, as well as examination of surgical pathology and autopsy specimens, some of the basic principles of cell life began to surface. I am thankful to Dr. Lauren V. Ackerman for allowing me to work independently in my field of investigation.

I give credit to Mr. Cramer K. Lewis of the Department of Illustration, Washington University School of Medicine, for the first eight black and white photomicrographs, taken in 1957 and 1958, before I began to take my own photomicrographs.

From 1959 until 1965, I served as the Chief of Laboratory Service at the Veterans Administration Hospital in McKinney, Texas, and also as Clinical Assistant Professor at the University of Texas Southwestern Medical School in Dallas. At that time a part of my research study, which was carried out under a U.S. Government grant, concerned various growth processes of chick embryos followed at close intervals from a freshly fertilized state until the time of hatching. This project was selected because it allowed me to observe the histogenetic processes of various morphological structures in chick embryos and compare my observations with adult tissues, as well as with the findings of some early observers whose views served as the basis for many commonly held theories on histogenesis propagated through the years. It is noteworthy that several other early authors did not agree with some of the theories which became more or less established and commonly believed. Together with the study of embryonic tissues, I also studied a few short-term tissue culture materials and observed the diverse characteristics which different cells may take, defying the general belief in related histogenesis. Since 1965 I have been carrying out basic research in cell and tissue generation, differentiation and transformation in my own laboratory, Diagnostic and Cell Research Institute, Waco, Texas, which I founded and have been supporting financially.

I greatly appreciate the permission for reproduction given by the following editors and publishers of the my previously published articles: *British Journal of Cancer* (figs. 1-6), *The Journal of the Indian Medical Association* (figs. 7-8) and *The Journal of the American Medical Women's Association* (figs. 9-11).

I am highly indebted to Mrs. Barbara Hobbs, the head of the Library Department of the Waco Veterans Administration Hospital, and her staff for kindly obtaining for me many original references, a few of which were a century old.

Throughout my investigative career, many persons assisted me immensely in different ways. I gratefully acknowledge my indebtedness particularly to the following persons for their efforts in assisting in various experiments, keeping all the records, preparing beautiful slides, making valuable suggestions, collecting various data, and many other duties: Tutter Levinson, Dixie McGregor, Lois Grawe, Allen Casten, William Bunch, Karen Lion, Susan Vartdol, and Bernard Machovsky. Mr. Machovsky has been directly assisting me for many years in my research studies with technical help and valuable suggestions. In addition, Dr. Janya Martin, Michael Soto, Dan Browder and Mr. Machovsky were invaluable for their editorial assistance in preparation of this book. Without Dr. Martin's encouragement this book might never have been published.

Finally, I wish to express my heartfelt thanks and great appreciation to my husband, Dr. Hendley A. McDonald, who has been a source of encouragement all these years, and has willingly borne all the inconveniences resulting from his wife's deep desire to keep on studying the microscopic world of cell life.

Waco, Texas
1988

Hemprova G. McDonald, M. D.

TABLE OF CONTENTS

CHAPTER ONE

BLOOD AND BLOOD VESSEL FORMATION FROM
CARDIAC MUSCLE · 23

    Development of blood and vascular channels is demonstrated in adult cardiac muscle
in humans and animals (such as rabbits, rats, mice, and chickens), and also briefly
in embryonic cardiac muscle of humans and chicks. In addition, possible red cell
development is demonstrated by chick embryonic cardiac muscle in tissue culture.

CHAPTER TWO

CARDIAC MUSCLE IN CHRONIC ISCHEMIA:
  DIRECT TRANSFORMATION (METAPLASIA) INTO COLLAGEN FIBERS · · 36

> Transformation of striated myofibers into collagen fibers with narrow spindle-shaped nuclei.

CHAPTER THREE

CARDIAC MUSCLE IN ACUTE RHEUMATIC FEVER: DEGENERATION, TRANSFORMATION, ASCHOFF BODY FORMATION, REGENERATION, AND FIBROSIS · 42

Various degenerative processes, particularly cellular lysis, of cardiac muscle are found to be the primary insults of acute rheumatic fever. The origin of Aschoff cells (Type A, B and C) of Aschoff bodies follow respective pathways of cytogenesis from damaged muscle products. In addition, other cellular components of Aschoff bodies also arise from damaged muscle. Regeneration of cardiac muscle may occur following redifferentiation of lymphocyte-like dedifferentiated cells of myogenic origin. Some Aschoff bodies represent an abortive attempt or atypical regeneration of cardiac muscle fibers. Both Aschoff bodies and associated collagenous fibrous tissue originate from damaged muscle.

CHAPTER FOUR

DAMAGE AND TRANSFORMATION OF CARDIAC MUSCLE IN CORONARY OCCLUSION FROM A SINGLE CASE STUDY · 63

In coronary occlusion, coagulation necrosis of muscle fibers may be followed by the in-situ origin of various reactive cells—histiocytes, 'phagocytes', plasma cells, lymphocytes, segmented nuclear cells, spindle cells, and many unclassified cells—as well as blood and blood capillaries towards the development of granulation tissue and fibrosis. Acute inflammatory exudate and 'hemorrhage' (linked with occasional cardiac rupture) show their origin from ischemic muscle. The development of small and large blood vessels from ischemic muscle is presented as a basis for collateral circulation.

Introduction

From the 1950's the author has noticed, as did many others, that in tissue sections many cellular structures cannot be categorized according to the well-known classification of cells. Subsequent zealous studies of many of these previously unexplained structures, whether in cellular forms or otherwise, has provided some understanding about them as the missing links in the continuous processes of cellular life. These basic processes include cell generation, differentiation, growth, transformation, dissolution, dedifferentiation, and redifferentiation into the same or different types of cells or tissues.

The results of the author's critical studies on the histogenesis of various cellular and tissue structures have been presented in annual sessions of various scientific organizations (Abstracts - McDonald 1957, 1958, 1961, 1962a, 1962b, 1962c, 1963b, 1970a, 1975b, 1975c, 1981, 1984, 1986). Her findings are also published as full articles in several national and international scientific journals (McDonald 1959a, 1959b, 1962d, 1963a, 1968, 1970b, 1975a, 1983, and McDonald and Calkins 1978). In 1989 the first volume of this present series appeared; in that volume various cytogenesis pathways in development of different morphological structures are explained. Both benign and malignant tissues are covered. Three of the above articles (1963b, 1975a, 1978) which are related to cardiac muscle in rheumatic fever are reproduced in their entirety in this volume as an appendix.

The vast amount of data that the author has accumulated on the cardiac muscle impels her to present them in a separate volume in this series. To demonstrate the broad scope of this study, in addition to the myocardium of humans, the myocardium of a few animals, such as rabbits, rats, mice and chicks, are also presented. These animals were used by the author in various short-term scientific experiments. In addition, this volume briefly demonstrates the embryonic development of human and chick cardiac muscle, as well as the cardiac muscle of chick embryos in tissue culture.

The first chapter of this volume deals with blood and blood vessel formation directly from cardiac muscle fibers of humans and animals. The direct development of red cells as hemoglobin globules is shown briefly in human and chick embryonic cardiac muscle fibers and also in the tissue culture product of the latter. The development of endothelium as well as smooth muscle coat of larger vessels is also shown to be of cardiac muscle origin.

The second chapter describes the mechanism of fibrosis of cardiac muscle fibers in gradual ischemic conditions. Here the cardiac muscle fibers directly transform into collagenous fibrous tissue with spindle-shaped nuclei. Such an occurrence is in contradiction to the pivotal role of fibroblasts, supposedly derived from embryonic mesenchymal lineage. (Other ways of development of fibrous tissue from cardiac muscle are described in the third and fourth chapters.)

The third chapter illustrates the damage of cardiac muscle and its subsequent reaction in the acute rheumatic fever disease process. This disease, which primarily affects the hearts of children, is now known to be a sequel of repeated Group A Streptococcus infection of the throat. Acute rheumatic fever was selected because the author's continued and detailed microscopic study of rheumatic hearts favors cardiac muscle damage and not the damage of collagen as the main culprit. This disease was the cause of death of many children before the advent of antibiotics. The author, personally, had the experience of seeing children die of cardiac failure in acute rheumatic fever in the early 1940s. The unique findings of this study are: 1. Acute rheumatic fever causes severe damage to the cardiac muscle with prominent cellular lysis and to a lesser extent fibrinoid and hyalin degenerations of cardiac muscle. 2. The unique cellular proliferation and the origin of fibrinoid material from damaged muscle as well as from regenerating myoplasm (which also gives the appearance of fibrinoid material in H&E stain) are involved in the mechanism for the production of Aschoff bodies, the diagnostic feature of rheumatic fever. 3. Even in fatal cases there is ample evidence of regeneration of cardiac muscle without mitosis. (This is accomplished by redifferentiation of dedifferentiated cells arising in lytic myofibers.) 4. The production of collagen fibers in the development of myocardial scar tissue is found to be the consequence of muscle damage and inadequate muscle regeneration. 5. Finally, the acute inflammatory infiltrate that often occurs in cardiac valves is shown to be of local origin, either from cardiac muscle or from myogenic fibrous tissue of cardiac valves.

In the fourth chapter on acute myocardial infarction, a variety of ways in which cardiac muscle in various stages of coagulation necrosis attempts recovery by development of fibrous tissue are described. Towards this goal the affected muscle fibers may transform into granulation tissue with production of blood capillaries and different types of inflammatory or reactive cells. Also, infarcted muscle may transform into collagenous fibrous tissue either directly or via chronic reactive cells of muscle origin. The massive generation of acute inflammatory cells (primarily segmented nuclear cells) of muscle origin associated with the destruction of muscle fibers, usually known as acute myocarditis, is known to be one of the two primary causes of the rupture of the cardiac wall in acute myocardial infarction. The second cause, which is known as hemorrhage in the cardiac wall, is actually found to be massive generation of blood by the freshly infarcted muscle fibers.

A brief summary of Volume I of *New Concepts in Blood Formation and Cell Generation in Malignant and Benign Tissues* (McDonald 1989) is given below so that one may be familiarized with some of the author's additional observations on histocytogenesis in various tissues and organs.

The mechanism of development of various epithelial patterns in breast carcinomas with emphasis on active cellular lysis as a means of acquiring space and nutrients for future growth and development of various epithelial patterns is briefly described; for more details see McDonald (1959a).

Examples are given of direct development of red cells as hemoglobin globules like secretion globules from local benign tissues include renal epithelium, liver parenchyma, epidermis, dermis, gastric mucosa and muscle coat, adipose tissue, collagen fibers, all three types of muscle fibers (skeletal, cardiac and smooth), and various cellular elements of the spleen.

Along with the formation of red cells, the development of endothelial membrane enclosing columns of formative red cells and the original plasma (liquified tissue product) has been demonstrated in various benign and malignant tissues.

Hemoglobin globules may also be formed by inflammatory or reactive cells: neutrophils, segmented nuclear cells (SN cells), lymphocytes, eosinophils, plasma cells, endothelial cells, and less well-defined cells as monocytes and histiocytes/phagocytes. Local origin of these reactive cells is demonstrated in benign and malignant tissues. Plasma cells may produce other types of inflammatory or reactive cells having erythrogenic capacity such as Russell body cells, segmented nuclear cells, neutrophils, eosinophils, lymphocytes and histiocytes.

Malignant tissues (including mammary carcinoma in humans and in mice, basal cell carcinoma, squamous cell carcinoma, colon carcinoma, renal carcinoma, prostatic carcinoma, and malignant melanomas in human and dog) demonstrate their erythrogenic capacity directly, as well as their capacity to produce various reactive cells and collagenous fibrous tissue also with erythrogenic capacity.

Development of red cells as hemoglobin globules from liquified tissue product particularly that of malignant tissues is demonstrated. According to the morphological characteristics, this tissue has been named plasma gel when the fluid product is clear and colorless, erythrogenic gel when it is red-sheded, and hemoglobin gel when it stains like concentrated hemoglobin. Prominent in malignant tissue is the formation of often vacuolated mesh-like structure prior to red cell formation. This structure has been named by the author as erythrogenic mesh. Acellular bone marrow fluid (in clot section) also shows a large number of red cells developing through this stage of erythrogenic mesh and erythrogenic gel.

Colorless hamolysis of red cells (figs. 138 and 139, Vol. I) in circulating blood, bone marrow and various tissues is believed by the author to be the normal way of removal of aged and defunct red cells. This is probably the mechanism that occurs in autoimmune hemolytic anemia. What would otherwise be considered erythrophagocytosis as a means for removal of aged red cells is shown by the author to actually be intracellular development of red cells.

Finally the different ways and different sources involved in the development of red cells are presented in a diagram, which is reproduced from Vol. I, on page 19.

It is important to refer to the history of different ways of red cell formation (in agreement with the author's observations) as found by early researchers; and also, how Neumann's commonly believed theory of only one specific way of nucleated erythropoiesis occurring only in bone marrow was more or less established. Weber and Kölliker (1845) followed the origin of red blood corpuscles in the cytoplasm of liver cells. Jones (1846) and Drummond (1854) both asserted that nucleated colorless cells (white blood cells) can produce red blood corpuscles without passing through a series of transitional stages. Wedl (1853) observed non-nucleated red blood cell formation in human cancers and normal tissues. Rollet (1862) and Rindfleisch (1863) maintained that red blood corpuscles arise as non-nucleated offspring of other cells as secretory globules. Heitzmann (1872) believed that protoplasm of hematoblastic substance can break into fragments which are themselves formed into red blood corpuscles. Ranvier (1874) and Schaeffer (1874) observed the origin of red blood corpuscles through endogenous intraprotoplasmic differentiation of vasoformative cells. Similarly, the unicellular origin of red cells with surrounding endothelial lining was observed by Sabin (1920). She named the mother cells angioblasts. Latta (1921) noted red blood corpuscle formation in the connective tissue of the intestine. Jordan (1926) described transformation of lymphocytes directly into erythrocytes.

By applying various diagnostic tools, Keasby (1923) concluded that hemoglobin is present in the globules of the globular leukocytes (same as Russell body cells or grape cells) derived from plasma cells. Duran Jorda described secretion-like origin of red blood cells (1947) and origin of red blood cells from eosinophils (1948). Neumann wrote many papers concerning one specific way of nucleated erythropoiesis as the only way of red cell formation, beginning in 1868, as mentioned by Michels (1931). Neumann propounded the theory that throughout mammalian life, red blood corpuscles arise only through one distinctive series of nucleated phases which occur exclusively in the bone marrow in adult life. Numerous authors have disagreed with Neumann's theory. Michels stated that, owing partly to the tenacity with which Neumann held to his views and to the strength with which he opposed all others, his theory had great impact. Michels also stated that one investigator, Robin (1874), claimed that Neumann's theory was actually "encumbering science."

The title of this work, *New Concepts in Blood Formation and Cell Generation,* is intended to represent a widely inclusive series of processes which are active throughout human and animal life forms. These concepts, based on investigations made and being made, will be presented in a series of books, the first of which considers several solid malignant tumors together with a few examples from benign tissues as mentioned above. Future volumes will discuss a few additional malignant tumors, and various benign tissues and organs, including bone marrow and circulating blood, for even in the latter there is evidence of cell generation and cell differentiation.

The author is aware of the fact that all her concepts in cell generation are not new, as a few basic findings on red cell formation were observed by early researchers; some of these references are over a century old, as stated above. Somehow these important findings were overshadowed by some influential authors; now, even as historical information, they are not mentioned in easily available books and journals, and therefore remain unknown. In this regard, "new concepts" for the title may be justified.

I. Red Cell Formation Directly as Hemoglobin Globules from Malignant and Benign Tissues, Including Reactive (Inflammatory) Cells

As demonstrated in this book from various organs and tissues and from reactive cells, the developmental processes of red cells without passing through the nucleated phases of erythropoiesis, as generally believed to be the only way of red cell formation

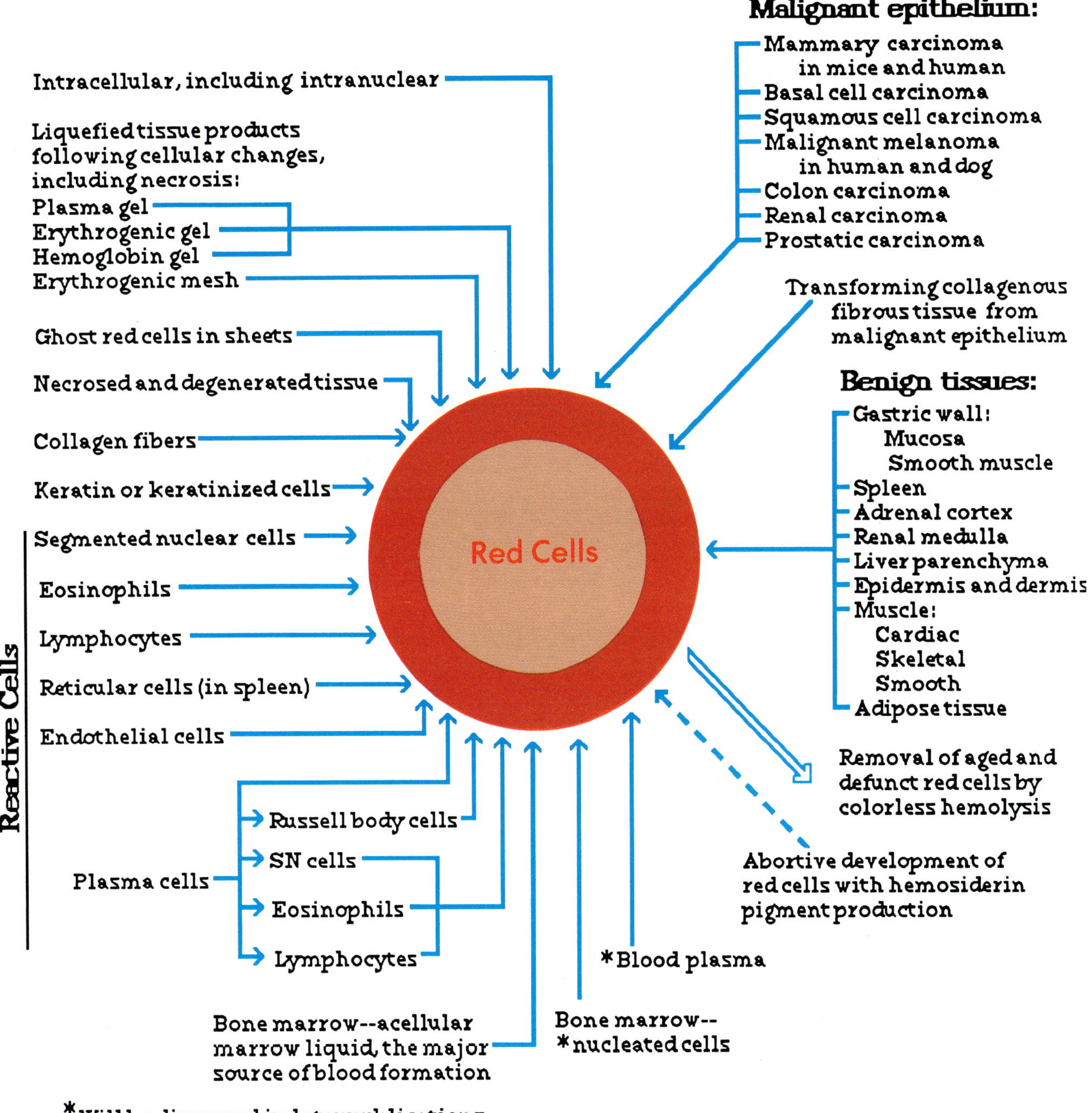

Author's note: This diagram is reproduced from Volume I (McDonald 1989) to demonstrate the variety of ways and different sources involved in the development of red blood cells.

Preconsiderations on the Approach of Study

Cellular study using tissue sections is found to be an excellent way to follow the natural biological processes in the development of various histological structures. Le Gross-Clark (1958) remarked that in tissue sections with simple stain, histological processes can be studied when the cellular structures are not dissociated. In addition to the microscopic examination of tissue sections, critical examinations of many photomicrographs have proven to be very helpful. With an analytical mind, careful and repeated examinations of photomicrographs, hours of 'groping' usually result in the discovery of missing links, however incomplete they may be, in the cellular and tissue growth processes.

The author would like to emphasize the fact that our present day technology, remarkable as it is, often helps us overlook the obvious. We should not let ourselves over-rely on technology and curtail our power of observation and analysis using our greatest tool: the human mind.

Preconceived ideas and beliefs on various histologic processes apparently limit one's accurate view of the phenomenon at hand and cause findings, which may be a part of the developmental processes, to be ignored. There is much to be learned about the capacity of the living substance for cell generation, differentiation and transformation. Based on circumstantial evidence William E. Horner, Professor of Anatomy at the University of Pennsylvania, pointed out in his book *Special Anatomy and Histology* (1851), the possibility of the development of new elements, in the laboratory of animal systems inside the body, by the all-controlling influence of living principle. One must experience an aura of wonder when he or she tries to imagine the complexity, intricacy and diversity of the enormous biochemical reactions that must be taking place in order to transform the simple looking white and yellow of a fertilized egg into a fully developed chick embryo with feathers, a brain, and everything else, while still within the shell. It would not be out of place to suspect that there may be many new elements, as well as additions to the existing known elements, created by the all-controlling influence to build this fully developed embryo.

The cell patterns seen at one point only identify the characteristics for that time, as there is a continuous process of cell differentiation often in different directions and at different speeds. The nucleus, cytoplasm, cell membrane, and intercellular substances are all forming, transforming or dissolving in a continuous protoplasmic mass from which

similar or completely different kinds of cells and tissue structures may make their appearance, as suggested in this book and in the author's previous publications.

The author is aware of the fact that there must be many gaps not yet considered in her description of various cellular changes. She hopes that with these preliminary findings, further studies by inquisitive minds will unveil additional pathways of cellular and tissue growth, the full extent of which is beyond human capability.

The preconceived idea that every cell has to come from similar cells of embryological lineage and through mitosis has prevented the understanding of cellular and tissue growth patterns to a great extent. Schwann (1847), who made a classical study on cells over a century ago, pointed out the difficulties in formulating any scheme for the classification of cells of different histological structures:

> Nature is very unwilling to accommodate herself to our schemes. The object of her aim is quite opposed to that of our intellect. She accords and accommodates all contrarieties by gentle transition: the intellect disjoins and seeks everywhere for strongly marked contrast.

The classic description of cells may fit at certain stages of development, but there are many more cells present in tissue sections which do not conform to our classification. One must remember that tissue sections represent the cross sections of dynamic growth processes in various stages of development in a natural setting. The author's mode of study conforms with that of Weiss (1950) who stated,

> we must form the habit . . . of viewing the shape of a given cell, tissue, or organ not as a static feature, but as a phase, transitory or terminal, in a continuous chain of transformation: as a cross section through a stream of processes proceeding in time. Every morphological criterion is but an expression of antecedent processes that have contributed to its formation.

This habit of study also calls for inquiry into the possible future development from the present status of cells and tissues in view.

In this book and in earlier publications the author has been trying to show her microscopic findings of "gentle transition" in the development of the different cellular and tissue structures guided by nature.

Materials and Methods of Study

For this study of cardiac muscle, sections were taken mainly from the left ventricular wall or interventricular septum of humans and animals (rabbits, rats, and mice). The human cardiac tissues were obtained mainly from relatively fresh autopsy specimens except for two figures which were taken from the original heart of a patient that had undergone a heart transplant. The myocardium of a few human embryos, the products of miscarriages, were studied as well as chick embryos and chick embryonic cardiac muscle grown in tissue culture media. In connection with the author's experimental chemotherapy program using C3H mice with spontaneous or transplanted breast carcinomas, many hearts were examined for detection of possible metastasis (McDonald 1959a). It is interesting to note that cardiac muscle, especially that of mice, is completely resistant to metastasis by mammary carcinoma. In several instances there are large, freely growing metastatic tumor emboli filling the right ventricular cavity and pressing against the cardiac wall to the point of rupture. Still there is no evidence for tumor intake by the cardiac muscle in the invasion of muscle wall (McDonald 1959a).

Other animals were used in relation to the author's different short-term experimental projects. The myocardium of rats was examined in relation to toxicology testing. Rabbits were used to study blood regeneration following the heavy loss of blood.

In addition to the microscopic study of tissue sections, hundreds of related photomicrographs have been critically examined and analyzed in order to learn the relationships among various cellular and tissue structures concerning dedifferentiation, transformation, and regeneration. Repeated examinations of the same photomicrographs or tissue slides often revealed additional findings which were not recognized upon earlier examinations.

Demonstrations made by these photomicrographs are based mainly on light microscopic study of 10% neutral formalin-fixed tissues. (The tissues of rheumatic fever cases of the 1930's and 1940's have been fixed in Zenker-formol solution.) Occasionally phase contrast microscopy was used. Tissues were sectioned at four to six micron thickness and stained routinely with hematoxylin and eosin (H&E) stain. Sections were also frequently stained with Giemsa stain, and when indicated for detection of iron pigment, Prussian blue reaction was tested. Some sections were studied with the application of a battery of special histochemical stains such as Mallory's phosphotungstic acid hematoxylin, Mallory's aniline blue-acid fuchsin orange G, Verhoeff van Gieson stain, Masson's trichrome stain, Foot's modification of Bielschowsky's method for reticulum stain, periodic acid Schiff method of McManus, and Benhold's Congo red stain. For confirmation of shapes of certain morphological structures in their entirety in three dimensions, serial sections were examined in a few instances.

NOTES

CHAPTER ONE
BLOOD AND BLOOD VESSEL FORMATION
FROM CARDIAC MUSCLE

Development of blood and vascular channels is demonstrated in adult cardiac muscle in humans and in animals (such as rabbits, rats, mice, and chickens), and also briefly in embryonic cardiac muscle of humans and chicks. In addition, possible red cell development is demonstrated by chick embryonic muscle in tissue culture media.

I. INTRODUCTION

The possibility that practically all tissues (in addition to bone marrow) have the potential for generation of blood, vascular channels, and a variety of inflammatory or reactive cells has been studied by the author for many years. Such capacities by many organs and tissues, including malignant tissues, are presented with color photomicrographs and summarized by charts and diagrams in Vol. I of this series (McDonald 1989).

This first chapter deals with blood and vascular channel formation from cardiac muscle fibers of humans and animals. Various ways of red cell formation associated with the development of original plasma and endothelial lining of vascular channels (all from cardiac muscle) are discussed in this chapter. There is a strong suggestion that the smooth muscle coat and adventitia of the vessel wall are also of cardiac muscle origin. The mechanism of elongation and widening of vascular channels is explained in this chapter. Finally, a brief background on the vital phenomenon of cellular lysis in various aspects of growth processes is presented (McDonald 1959b, 1962d, 1975a and 1989).

II. DEVELOPMENT OF RED CELLS

1. Direct development as hemoglobin globules from cardiac muscle

The most common way of red cell generation from cardiac muscle fibers (and also from other organs and tissues) is the direct development of hemoglobin globules. Morphologically, this process may be compared to the development of secretion globules or inclusion bodies. Usually the red cells are developed as round bodies of regular size, similar to red blood cells of circulating blood, as illustrated in figures 1-3, but occasionally marked variation in size and shape may be seen (fig. 4).

Red cells do not necessarily originate as round bodies, but may instead initially appear as a stack of rectangular blocks lying in columns (figs. 11-1, 11-2 and 12). These rectangular red cells eventually develop into regularly shaped red cells when they lie in a fluid medium after being dislodged from the surrounding muscle element.

Also arising in muscle, red cells may start as hyalin globules (fig. 5) or granules of broken altered muscle substance (fig. 11-2). (See also fig. 37-2.) The latter occurence is frequently observed to occupy irregular areas of muscle under acute stressful, anoxic conditions as shown in figure 11-2. A similar way of red cell formation in development of a large blood vessel is shown in ischemic cardiac muscle in acute myocardial infarction (fig. 87). How quickly and extensively this way of blood for-

mation may take place under extremely stressful conditions is demonstrated in the liver by figure 13-1 (this is a reproduction of figure 127-1, Vol. I). This figure shows a large, expanding blood vessel with tributaries, developing from liver parenchyma (undergoing fragmentation and granulation) in less than an hour's time. Similar observations in red cell formation in the liver were made over a century ago by Weber and Kolliker (1845). Heitzmann (1872) also believed that protoplasm of hematoblastic substances can break into fragments which form into red blood corpuscles themselves.

The presence of red cells outside the blood vessels (fig. 11-2) is commonly mistaken for 'hemorrhage' even though there is no evidence of tissue compression or any other type of distortion. Also there are no ruptured vessels, no evidence of trauma, and no scattered blood cells overlying the normal tissue. The lack of these evidences rules out the possibility of hemorrhage.

Hemoglobin concentration may vary in developing red cells. Some red cells may have very little hemoglobin and may be categorized as ghost red cells or markedly hypochromatic red cells. Others may be fully, or even hyper-hemoglobinized as suggested by their staining characteristics (figs. 1-4). Sometimes developing red cells may even appear as hyalin globules from muscle fibers (arrows, fig. 5).

Usually, red cells arise in a single column along the longitudinal plane of the muscle fibers in the development of narrow blood capillaries (figs. 1, 4, 11 and 12). In the development of larger capillaries wider columns of red cells, sometimes occupying the whole thickness of one or more muscle fibers, may be formed (figs. 2, 3 and 5). The direction of the developing red cell column may change and cross the myofiber or myofibers, probably in anticipation of anastomosis with other blood capillaries, figure 1 (A).

2. Development of red cells through intermediary reactive cells—most commonly segmented nuclear cells (SN Cells)—of muscle origin

In addition to the most common way of red cell formation, i.e., direct development of hemoglobin globules from myoplasm, a few red cells may develop from intermediary reactive or inflammatory cells of cardiac muscle origin even in apparently normal muscle (figs. 6 and 11-3). These erythrogenic reactive cells may develop in columns toward the formation of blood capillaries. Many examples are given in chapter four of red cell development from different reactive cells (SN cells, lymphocytes, eosinophils, plasma cells, monocytes, and histiocytes) of cardiac muscle origin in acute myocardial infarction. Similar observations were made in several benign and malignant tissues in Vol. I. The usual tendency is to designate this phenomenon as erythrophagocytosis instead of erythrogenesis. These reactive cells are therefore commonly catagorized as erythrophagocytotic neutrophils, erythrophagocytotic lymphocytes, erythrophagocytotic histiocytes, etc. Such a conclusion was made by Listinsky (1988) in her report that in 23 patients, auxillary node dis-

section revealed various degrees of erythrophagocytosis with or without prior trauma of breast biopsy. The author's observations on lymph nodes, which will be published in a future volume, suggest that there are many examples of red cell formation from various reactive cells. Similar cells with erythrogenic capacity are demonstrated in the spleen and other tissues in Vol. I. The author also demonstrates—in the adrenal gland, gastric wall, and breast cancers—the origin of columns of SN cells transforming into columns of red cells within the lumen areas of developing capillaries. A profuse number of erythrogenic SN cells are seen in bone marrow, in areas of acute inflammation, and in granulation tissue. The acceptance of the theory of erythrophagocytosis rather than erythrogenesis probably arises from the deep-rooted belief that extramedullary tissues have no erythrogenic capability, and that each erythrocyte must pass through the distinctive nucleated phases of erythropoiesis.

The stimulus for development of blood by cardiac muscle may vary greatly from one focal area to another (figs. 12 and 12-1). While the muscle shown in figure 12 reacted with marked blood and blood vessel formation, the nearby area (fig. 12-1) shows marked dissolution of cardiac muscle with production of wide clefts filled with apparently clear fluid. The extensive loss of myocardial tissue through lysis (fig. 36-1) is not often appreciated and may be termed as edema, or discarded as artifact caused by improper handling of the tissue section. This is exemplified in the chapter on acute rheumatic fever. Occasionally, red cells may develop via crystallization of hemoglobin gel (deep red liquified product in gel form, figure 13).

III. DEVELOPMENT OF PLASMA

Another important part of blood and vascular channel formation is the development of original plasma within newly formed blood vessels. (When no red cells are present in the lumen, the channel is commonly termed a lymphatic vessel.) The newly formed, locally derived red cells are soon separated from the remaining mother substance by clear and colorless liquefaction of the latter thus producing original plasma in the lumen. In figures 4, 5 and 12, the partial clearing of the developing capillary lumen is due to the formation of clear plasma. In the case of lymphatic channels, the entire lumen is filled with plasma although a few red cells may be seen occasionally.

In contrast to skeletal muscle, cardiac muscle becomes liquefied more easily and forms wide clefts, which are often interconnected and filled with clear fluid (fig. 12-

1). When lined by endothelium such clefts are commonly termed lymphatic channels (figs. 34, 37). Such observations led Cowdry (1950) to conclude the existence of the profuse lymphatic drainage of cardiac muscle in contrast to skeletal muscle. The presence of such lymphatic channels is more abundant where lysis of cardiac muscle is prominent. A similar way of lymphatic channel formation usually without lymphocytes in the lumen can be seen in practically all tissues. The importance of such a mechanism in vessel formation is emphasized in cancer because undissolved tumor tissue lying in the vascular lumen may act as a source of metastasis.

Developing processes of a lymphatic channel containing lymphocytes in the lumen can be seen in figure 10. The channel and its contents (lymph plasma and lymphocytes) all arise from the lysing cardiac muscle within the lumen area of the developing lymphatic vessels. This process of development of lymphatic channels with lymphocytes is common in lymphoid tissues; lymphocytes arise as small, round, hyperchromatic nuclei.

IV. DEVELOPMENT OF ENDOTHELIUM AND SMOOTH MUSCULAR COAT OF VASCULAR WALL

The origin of endothelium usually takes place from the peripheral remaining muscle element enclosing red cell columns (or columns of plasma) as demonstrated in figures 1-5, 7, 8, 10, 11 and 15. In this exanguated original heart of a cardiac transplant patient, the developing process of vascular channels through cellular lysis and the development of the endothelial lining and a surrounding smooth muscle layer are demonstrated in figures 7-9.

The progressive development of smooth muscle coat from the loose fibrous element of cardiac muscle origin (peripheral to endothelium) is shown in figures 7, 8 and 9. This process includes the progressive development of tiny, linearly placed, dedifferentiated cells expanding in a creeping manner followed by their redifferentiation into smooth muscle coat of the vessel wall. These cells are somewhat similar to lymphocytes and arise from cardiac muscle or myogenic connective tissue.

V. THE MECHANISM OF LENGHTENING AND WIDENING OF VASCULAR CHANNELS

Lenghtening of blood vessels may occur by the extension of morphological changes similar to the ones described above for independent blood vessel formation. The lengthening of the vessel may also occur by joining the ends of independently developed capillaries. Tiny independent primordia of blood vessels may originate as small, round, vascular units which are close to each other. Unification of these units by dissolution of the intervening cell substance lengthens the capillary. These tiny vascular units lying close to each other and in a line may be formed of single cells (fig. 21) or multiple cells (fig. 22).

The mechanism of widening the girth of blood vessels occurs by the dissolution of existing walls and immediate peripheral adjacent tissue (whether the latter is forming blood or not) followed by the re-establishment of a new vascular wall. By doing so, the emerging blood vessel has quickly enhanced its capacity to hold the larger blood column as shown in figure 13-1 in the liver.

The author agrees with the findings of Clark and Clark (1932) who observed blood capillary development in the rabbit ear and stated, "There is evidence to show that under stable conditions new capillaries are continually being formed while others may be retracted and absorbed, so that the capillary pattern in any part of the body is plastic and capable of alteration from time to time in response to changes in the immediate environment."

The popular theory concerning the origin of vascular channels is that, "After the closed vascular system has developed in the embryo and the circulation begun, new blood vessels always arise by 'budding' from pre-existing blood vessels", (Maximow and Bloom, 1957). As evidenced in this chapter and earlier publications, the author's findings advocate the concept of independent origin of vascular channels from local tissues. This process of independent development was observed by Wedl (1853) within the parenchyma of cancer and in exudation undergoing organization. The independent origin of blood and blood vessels is shown by the author in many organs and tissues, benign and malignant, in the first volume. The author's earlier publications support the origin of vascular channels from breast cancer tissue (McDonald 1962d) and from liver parenchyma (McDonald 1968).

VI. CELLULAR LYSIS: A PHENOMENON OF GROWTH PROCESSES

Due to its essential role in the development of vascular channels in addition to other developmental processes it is important to briefly discuss the phenomenon of cellular lysis. As shown in the author's previous publications, cellular lysis is an important aspect of growth processes of various morphological structures in benign and malignant tissues

(McDonald 1959b, 1962d, 1968, 1989). As Shaver (1953) suggested, cellular lysis provides the space and fluid containing the vital substances (self-reproducing enzymes) for the origin and growth of new cells. In benign tissues, this process proceeds less visibly, and is difficult to see unless one examines the tissue sections critically. In malignant tissues the lytic process is usually obvious (more so in some tumors than in others). The main cellular changes leading to cell lysis are observed and categorized by the author as cell digestion (such as liquefied by proteolytic enzymes), hydropic degeneration (watery, vacuolar changes), and other changes including tissue necrosis. Necrosis, which is not usually seen in benign tissues unless diseased, is common in malignant tumors. The faster the rate of cell generation, the more rapid is the lytic process. New growth out of digested or necrosed tissues is commonly observed in cancers with development, as well as interchanging of various epithelial patterns McDonald (1959b). The contribution of cellular lysis to the formation of vascular contents in malignant and benign tissues has been shown over three decades. There are also many examples of blood vessel formation

initiated by cellular lysis shown in various organs and tissues in Vol. I of this series (McDonald 1989).

The role of lysis of cardiac muscle in the development of new vascular channels in myocardium was explained earlier in this chapter. Lysis of myofibers creates vascular spaces and original plasma. The lytic product may also produce red cells directly as hemoglobin globules (fig. 13). Extensive lysis of cardiac muscle resulting in the development of large clefts or sinuses containing clear fluid, which is commonly called edema fluid, is shown in acute rheumatic fever in the third chapter. If these clefts or sinuses are lined by endothelium the fluid is known as plasma (lymph plasma or blood plasma) and the channels are called lymphatic vessels or blood vessels. It is conceivable that fragments of tissue destined for vessel formation may resist complete lysis and be carried away as emboli. Lie (1987) reported myocardial tissue fragments as emboli in the systemic and pulmonary circulation. The possibility of tumor tissue also resisting complete lysis and acting as a source of distant metastasis was discussed by the author in breast carcinomas (McDonald 1962d and 1989, p. 21).

VII. DEVELOPMENT RED CELLS FROM EMBRYONIC CARDIAC MUSCLE IN HUMANS AND IN CHICKS; AND DEVELOPMENT OF RED CELLS AND FAT GLOBULES FROM EMBRYONIC CARDIAC MUSCLE *IN VITRO*

In addition to the study of adult tissues, the direct development of red cells was also studied in embryonic tissues of humans and chicks. In the early part of the 1960s the author was involved in the study of embryonic tissues using chick embryos at short intervals during the incubation period. These studies were performed to learn more about the developmental processes of various morphological structures. Many embryos were serially sectioned at 5 microns and routinely stained with H&E stain and occasionally special stains were used. Many stained and unstained tissue sections have been carefully preserved for present and future study. Partial findings of this embryological study concerning origin of vascular channels from epithelial tissue of the liver was previously published (McDonald 1968).

One may notice that without going through the nucleated stages, red cells are developing directly as hemoglobin globules from embryonic cardiac muscle cells, as demonstrated in humans (figs. 14 and 14-1) and chicks (fig. 15). (Note: both normal adult and embryonic red cells of the chicken are nucleated.) Direct development of red cells from local tissues has been noticed in various adult organs and tissues as demonstrated in Vol. I and seen in the diagram earlier in this volume page 19.

This embryological study extended to the study of embryonic tissues grown in tissue culture media. The cells were grown in tissue culture chambers (Aloe Scientific Company cat. no. V59072) between round cover slips in monolayer. The tissue culture media used consisted of Eagle's basic medium with 10% horse serum. The media was inoculated with chick embryonic cardiac muscle. At the end of the designated period, the cover slips were removed and appropriately stained for microscopic examination. This is the first time the author is demonstrating a few interesting findings from the *in vitro* part of this study.

The possibility of direct development of red cells from chick embryonic cardiac muscle grown in tissue culture media is suggested in figures 16 and 16-1. *In vitro* embryonic chick cardiac muscle cells form intracellular red cells starting as tiny hemoglobin globules with a central pinpoint nucleus. Soon the newly developing red cells increase in volume as shown in figures 16 and 16-1.

It is interesting to note that the embryonic cardiac muscle *in vitro* also has the capacity to produce intracellular fat (figs. 16-2 and 16-3). The importance of this finding is the understanding that cells have the intrinsic capacity to produce fat whether supplied from the outside or not.

VIII. EXPLANATION OF FIGURES

Figures 1-10 were taken from human cardiac muscle. Figures 1-3 are from a two-hour post-mortem cardiac muscle of a 43-year-old man who died of widely spreading naso-pharyngeal carcinoma with terminal pulmonary emboli. (Figures 1-3 are reproductions of figures 135-137 of Vol. I.) Figure 4 shows a two-hour postmortem cardiac muscle of a 22-month-old child who died of acute bronchopneumonia. Figures 5 and 6 are taken from the apparently normal myocardium of the same heart with typical myocardial infarction occurring elsewhere and discussed in the fourth chapter of this volume. Figures 7-10 are from the exanguated cardiac muscle of the original heart of a patient who underwent cardiac transplantation. He was a 76-year-old male with hypertensive arteriosclerotic heart disease and cardiomegaly.

Figures 11 and 11-1 were obtained from the cardiac muscle of a healthy rabbit that was used as a normal control in a bleeding experiment. The animal was sacrificed by intravenous injection of air (air embolism). Figure 11-2 is from the cardiac muscle of another control rabbit sacrificed by administration of a lethal dose of ether. Figure 11-3 is from the interventricular septal cardiac muscle of a rabbit that was used in an experiment to study the effect of acute blood loss by withdrawing 30 cc of whole blood from the heart. This rabbit was sacrificed by intravenous injection of air.

Figures 12, 12-1 and 12-2 were obtained from the cardiac muscle of a rat that died of toxicity of ethyl hydrazine acetate hydrochloride used in an experimental cancer chemotherapy study.

Figure 13 is from the cardiac muscle of a mouse that was sacrificed two days after an experiment to study the effect of sublethal blood loss.

Figure 13-1 was taken from a fresh specimen of liver from a mouse that died within thirty minutes after a lethal injection, given inadvertantly, of an experimental drug, ethyl-hydrazine acetate hydrochloride.

Figures 14 and 14-1 were obtained from the myocardium of a miscarried human embryo weighing 7.8 grams (gestation period unknown).

Figure 15 is from the myocardium of a 6-day-old chick embryo.

Figures 16 and 16-1 were taken from the cardiac muscle of a 7-day-old chick embryo grown *in vitro* for 4 days and 6 days, respectively. Figures 16-2 and 16-3 were obtained from the cardiac muscle of a 12-day-old chick embryo grown *in vitro* 4 days and 8 days, respectively.

1. Origin of blood, blood capillaries, vessels with muscular coats, and lymphatic channels with lymphocytes from cardiac muscles in humans (figs. 1-10)

Development of red cells and blood capillaries, narrow (figs. 1-3), and large (figs. 2-3) from cardiac muscle fibers

Figure 1. These capillaries are identified by a single column of developing red cells, some of which are in the ghost red cell stage (red cells with hardly any hemoglobin). The arrows point to the segments of capillaries where endothelial nuclei are arising from the peripheral remaining myofibrils. The capillary at (A) is exhibiting extension in a curved line across the muscle fiber. This occurence is probably taking place in preparation for anastomosis with other capillaries. (B) points to regular cardiac muscle cell nuclei which are fading away in the sarcoplasm. H&E x 520

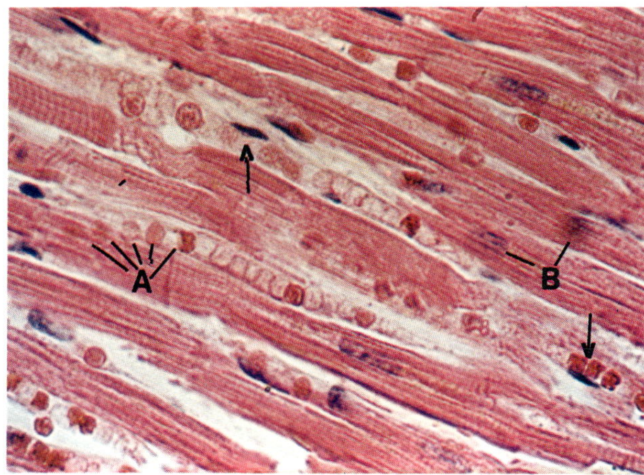

Figure 1

Figure 2. Forming out of the lysing muscle fibers, blood capillaries (A & B) contain developing red blood cells in early vacuolar stage. The wall of capillary (A) is formed by the outer rim of the remaining sarcoplasm (arrows), and the inner part of this wall is becoming endothelium with one endothelial nucleus in view. (C) is an obliquely cut small developing capillary. In a transverse plane, (D) are the narrowest developing capillaries with red cells in a single column. The arrows point to the remnants of lysing muscle which are becoming loose connective tissue between the muscle bundles. H&E x 520

Figure 3. Three large developing blood capillaries (A, B and C) of muscle cell origin in which the majority of the red cells are in the vacuolar stages (ghost red cell stage); however, a few are fully hemoglobinized. The right side of capillary (B) displays a partially developed endothelial membrane with one nucleus in view, while the blood column on the left side has not yet completely separated from the muscle fibers. Within capillary (C) red cells are developing from liquefying muscle elements. All these vessels are surrounded by developing endothelium of muscle origin. Upon close examination of blood vessels (A & C) the cross striations of vanishing muscle fibers are still visible (even in developing red cells). H&E x 520

Fully hemoglobinized red cells of various shapes and sizes arising along the longitudinal plane of the lysing muscle fibers (fig. 4)

Figure 4. Along the margin of a formative blood capillary, endothelial nuclei (A) and a partially formed endothelial membrane (arrow) are developing from muscle fibrils. (B) points to a muscle cell nucleus transforming into an endothelial nucleus. The newly formed red cells are mainly hyper-hemoglobinized and irregular in shape and size in contrast to developing red cells shown in figures 1-3. Note that along with dissolution of muscle element, the liquefied product (plasma) is seen in the vascular lumen as clear spaces. H&E x 575

Two completely different ways of red cell development from cardiac muscle: initial hyalin globular changes (fig. 5); and development of erythrogenic SN cells (fig. 6) (Figures 5 and 6 were taken from apparently normal cardiac muscle, away from the area of infarction, of a patient with recent myocardial infarction, presented in detail in chapter four)

Figure 5. Hyalin globular changes (arrows) are seen in cardiac muscle followed by hemoglobinization in the development of red cells. The columns of these red cells are developing into branching capillaries. (A) points to two endothelial nuclei arising in the lining muscle substance. H&E x 520

Figure 6. Scattered in this figure in irregular and regular columns are developing stages of erythrogenic segmented nuclear (SN) cells (arrows) derived from muscle fibers. The transformation stages of SN cells in production of hemoglobin (A), and then release of the hemoglobin as globules, i.e., red cells (B) into the lumen area of the developing blood capillary are seen here. At the end of the erythrogenic activity of SN cells, there is dissolution of the remaining cell substance in the developing blood plasma (see also figure 11-3). H&E x 520

Progressive developmental stages of smooth muscle coat of vascular channel arising from exanguated cardiac muscle undergoing fibrosis (figs. 7-9)

Figure 7. This figure demonstrates the development of three vascular channels (A, B and C), initiated by lysis of cardiac muscle fibers. Remnants of lysing muscle fibers are still evident in the lumens of vessels (A and C). The developing endothelium and endothelial nuclei from the lysing muscle element can be seen in this figure. In the left wall of channel (B) a line of tiny dedifferentiated nuclei are arising from changing cardiac muscle outside the developing endothelium. The progressive development of these nuclei continue in preparation for the formation of the smooth muscle coat of the vessel wall (this can be followed by the arrows in figures 7 to 9). H&E x 260

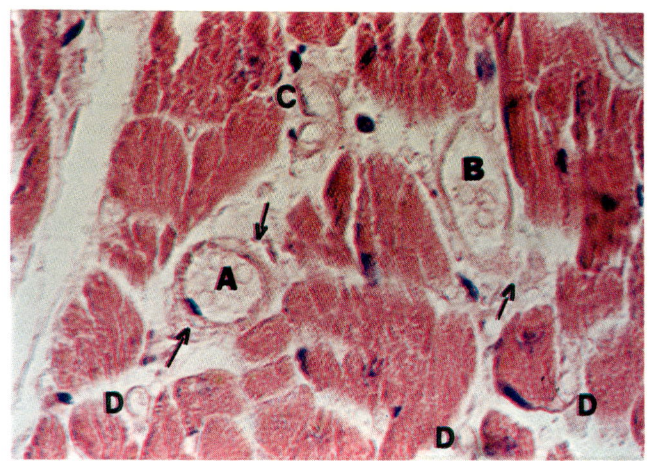

Figure 2

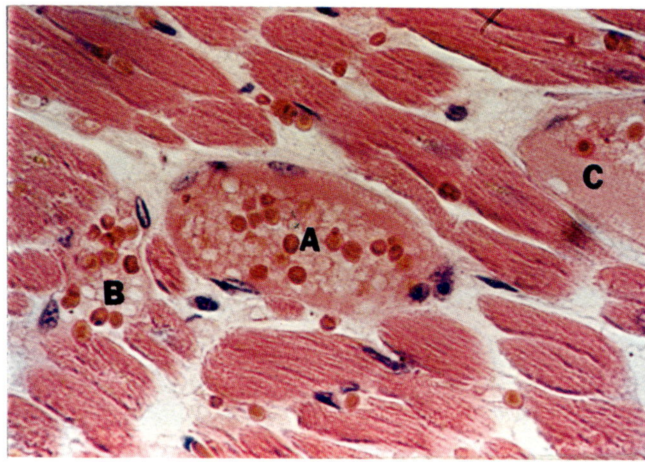

Figure 3

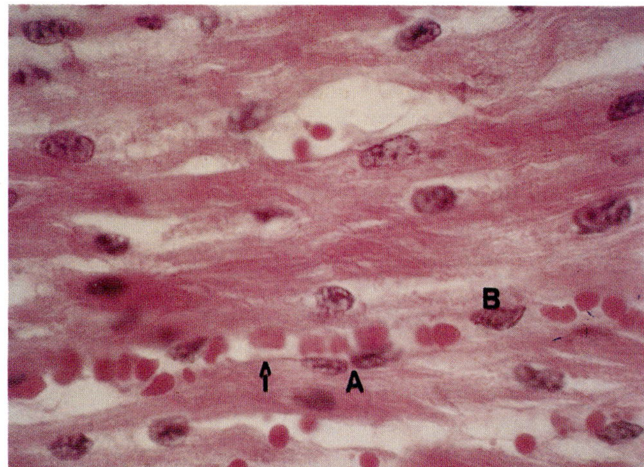

Figure 4

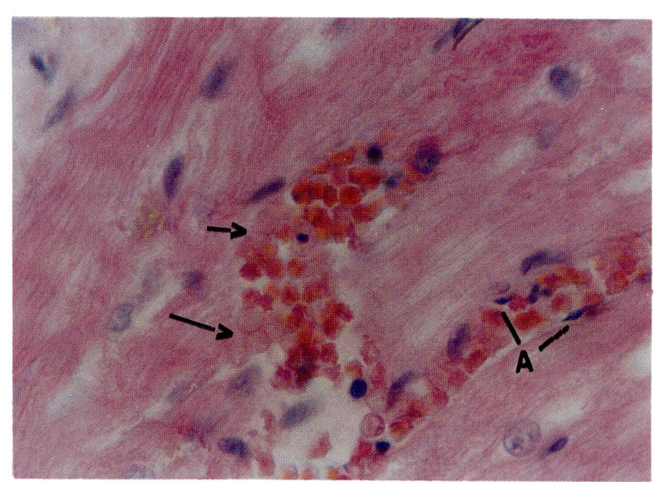

Figure 5

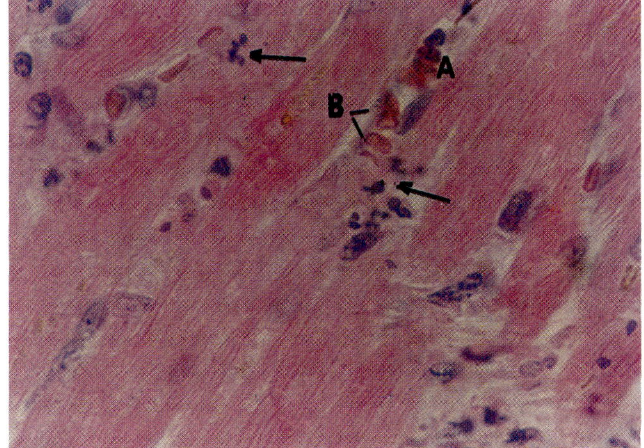

Figure 6

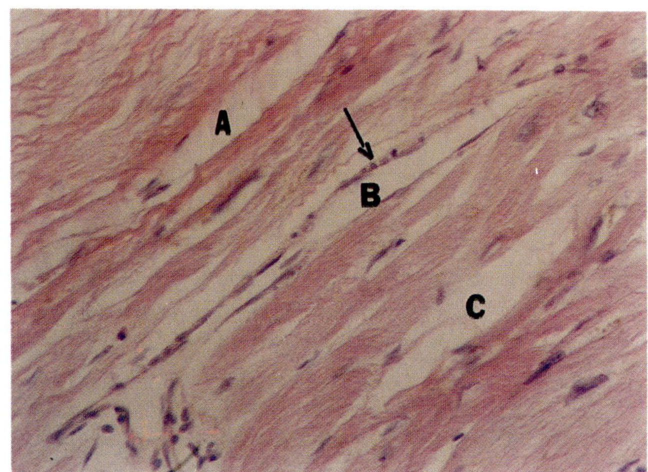

Figure 7

Figures 8 and 9. In addition to the development of smooth muscle coat there is a suggestion that adventitia also develops from myogenic loose connective tissue or even from liquefied muscle product. The capacity of the liquefied muscle element to give rise to new muscle as well as connective tissue fibers is shown in acute rheumatic fever. Figures 8 and 9, H&E x 260

Also from exanguated cardiac muscle, lymphatic channels and intra-luminal lymphocytes arising from liquefying cardiac muscle fibers (fig. 10)

Figure 10. Before their impending communication into a single vessel, (A and B) represent two adjoining developing lymphatic channels arising from the lysing cardiac muscle. (Note: at the site of their future communication, the intervening cell substance is dissolving.) The endothelial lining of channel (A) is partly formed, and three endothelial nuclei are in view. In developing channel (B), lymphocytes are arising from the liquefying muscle fibers. Some of the lymphocytes are situated in the lumen, and some others have not yet completely emerged from the liquefying muscle fibers shown at the edge. H&E x 520

2. Origin of blood and blood capillaries from cardiac muscles in rabbits (figs. 11 to 11-3)

Development of red cells and endothelium from cardiac muscle fibers in formation of narrow blood capillaries with single columns of red cells (figs. 11 and 11-1)

Figures 11 and 11-1. These red cells are originating as stacks of hemoglobin blocks in pressed-bisquit-type formation lying in single columns in longitudinal planes of cardiac muscle fibers. A magnified view of red cells in this formation can be seen in figure 11-1 (A). In figure 11, (A) points to a few endothelial nuclei arising from muscle fibers. Figure 11, H&E x 520; and figure 11-1, H&E x 1300

Rapid granular changes in cardiac muscle towards red cell development (fig. 11-2)

Figure 11-2. Under extreme stress, irregular foci of muscle tissue may undergo granular changes followed by hemoglobinization. Red cells are originating as fine, tiny,

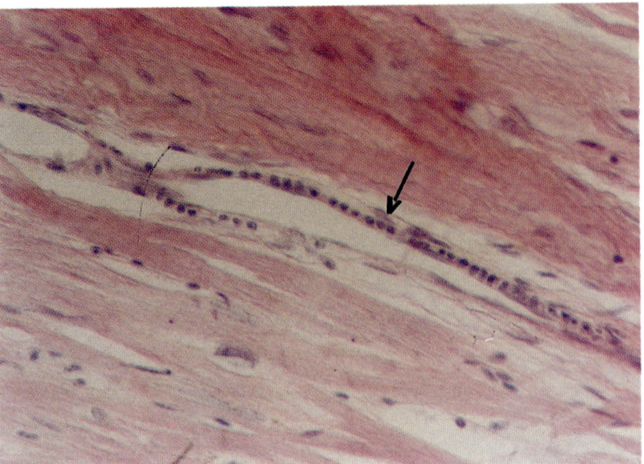

Figure 8

barely visible, reddish granules or particles (A) from disappearing muscle element. Continuous with (A) are areas of further development of hemoglobinized granules but not fully formed red cells (B). These developing red cells have fuzzy borders, as they are not yet completely free from the mother substance (the myoplasm). Casual observations of such findings as these are usually categorized as hemorrhage. For similar development of red cells within rapidly forming and expanding blood vessels from liver parenchyma see figure 13-1, and from ischemic cardiac muscle see figures 86 and 87. The arrow points to a narrow blood capillary containing similarly developing red cells. H&E x 130

Development of red cells from erythrogenic SN cells of muscle origin in formation of narrow blood capillaries (fig. 11-3)

Figure 11-3. (A's) point to two single columns of irregularly placed developing red cells (possibly developed through erythrogenic SN cells) still intimately connected with cardiac muscle element. The erythrogenic SN cells (B) lie within the course of a developing blood capillary of muscle fiber origin. Here also, red cells are not uniformly round and not placed in columns because of their irregular development from SN cells. (C) points to an erythrogenic cell that may be categorized as an erythrogenic lymphocyte. H&E x 520

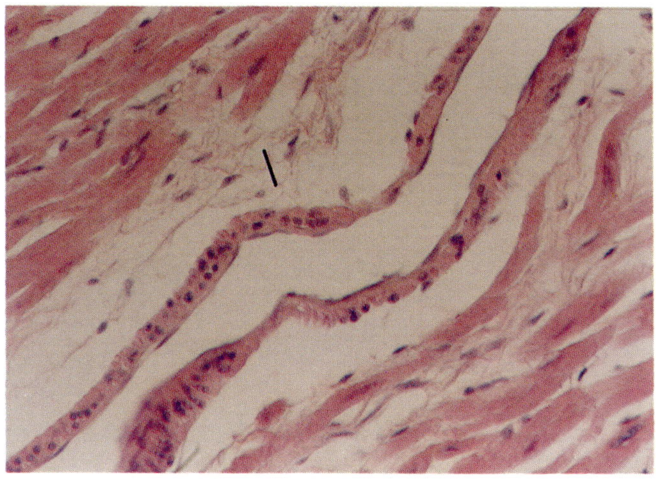

Figure 9

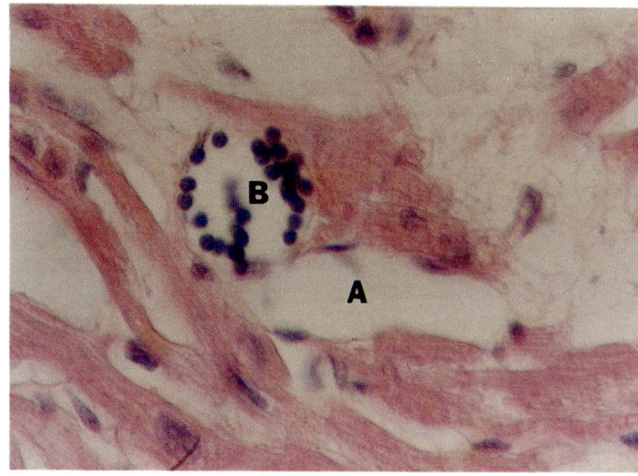

Figure 10

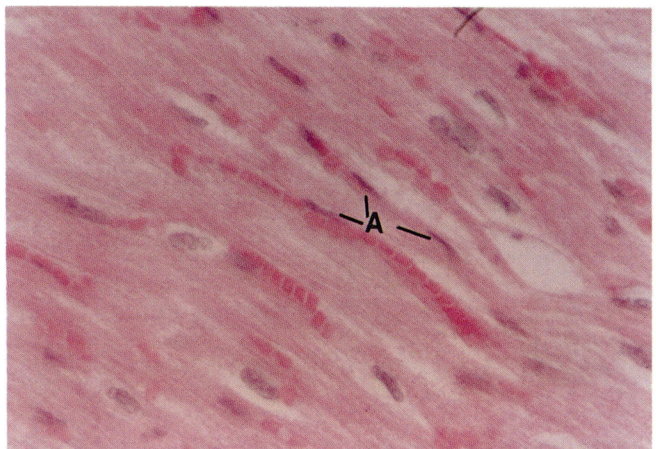

Figure 11

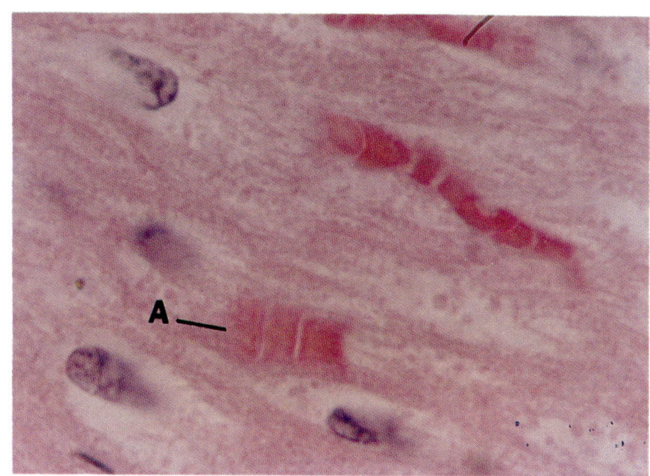

Figure 11-1

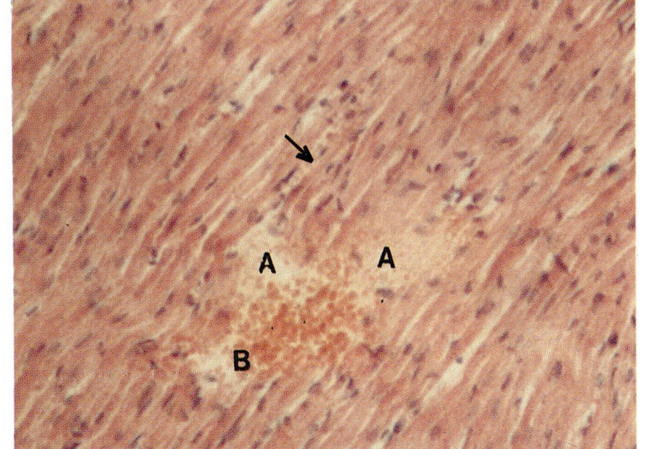

Figure 11-2

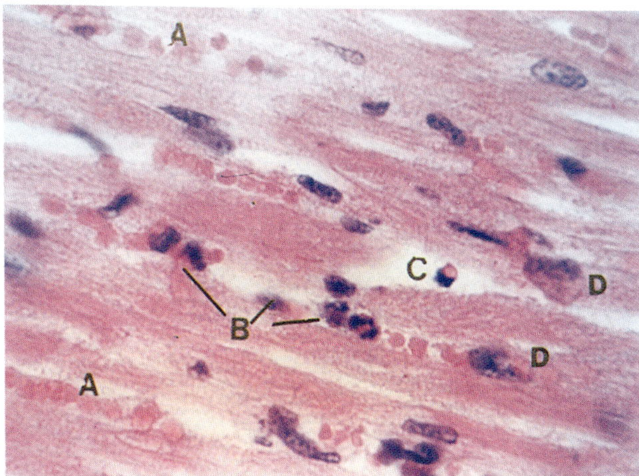

Figure 11-3

3. Origin of blood and vascular channels from cardiac muscle in rats (figs. 12 to 12-2)

(Figures 12 to 12-2 were taken from the same section of the myocardium of a rat, figure 12-2 is a higher magnification of a focal area of figure 12-1)

Profuse production of red cells mainly in single columns toward the development of many blood capillaries (fig. 12)

Figure 12. (a) points to an early stage and (b) to a later stage in the development of these red cells in a single column. (c) designates a large number of red cells (some which are not in columns) arising from cardiac muscles. The liquefaction of the remaining muscle substance within the developing capillaries contributes to the production of original plasma which is represented by the clear spaces in capillary (d) and other capillaries. The development of endothelial nuclei from myofibers is shown by (e) and (f). H&E x 80

Marked dissolution of cardiac muscle with production of wide, branching, cleft-like spaces filled with clear fluid of muscle lysis (figs. 12-1 and 12-2)

Figure 12-1. As opposed to figure 12, there is hardly any attempt for development of blood and blood vessels. Instead, myocardial lysis is producing wide cleft-like spaces filled with clear fluid commonly termed edema fluid or tissue fluid. Such fluid has been called lymph plasma when the channel is lined by endothelium (see figures 10, 34 and 37). From the lysing muscle fibers, two developing blood vessels (A and B) are also seen. H&E x 520

Figure 12-2. This is a magnified view of the developing blood vessel (B) and surrounding muscle shown in figure 12-1. Note that the red cells in the lumen are arising as hemoglobinizing fragments of muscle element; see also figure 37-3. H&E x 520

4. Origin of blood from cardiac muscle of a mouse (fig. 13)

A rare way of blood formation from hemoglobin gel produced by lysing cardiac muscle (fig. 13)

Figure 13. In these developing, communicating vascular channels, segment (A) is filled with deep red hemoglobin gel, and (B) points to developing red cells from hemoglobin gel, a process which may be called crystalization. (C) shows a compact, deformed red cell mass (the clear gap is artificially produced by tissue processing). (D) is probably in an earlier stage of development of compact deformed red cell mass from hemoglobin gel than (C). Compacting of the red cells is probably due to the high concentration of hemoglobin in hemoglobin gel. A magnifying glass will be helpful to study this figure. (Development of hemoglobin gel and of subsequent origin of deformed compact red cell masses are shown in breast carcinoma in figures 19, 33 and 33-1 in Vol. I.) H&E x 190

5. An example of how rapidly and extensively local tissue may transform into a large blood vessel packed with developing red cells, shown in liver parenchyma of a mouse (fig. 13-1)

Figure 13-1. This shows a large branching blood vessel rapidly developing from liver tissue undergoing granular fragmentation. Within this formative vascular channel not yet connected with the circulatory system, red cells are arising as angular hemoglobinized particles transformed from dissolving minute liver cell fragments (A). (B) liver cells lying in the path of vascular progression show similar early stages of red cell formation. (C) liver tissue at the periphery of the main vessel shows very early changes of red cell formation, and (C), on the left, points out the anticipated margin of further expansion of the vessel. (D) denotes endothelial nuclei of liver cell origin lining vascular wall. (E) shows early stages of endothelial nuclei development from liver cell nuclei. (F) red cells are originating in columns of one or more cells from liver parenchyma undergoing lysis in development of sinusoids. (Note: sinusoids are not usually lined by endothelium.) (G) liver cell nuclei are changing toward formation of lymphocytes. (H) multiple small nuclei, including those of lymphocyte size, are developing from liver cells. (I) at the upper right corner and near the center, the remains of liver cell nuclei are fading away in the cytoplasm. (J) shows lymphocytes developing from liver cells. (Note a few lymphocytes among the developing red cells in the lumen of the main vessel.) (K) endothelial nuclei and lymphocytes (at the margin of the vanishing vascular wall) are in the process of being transformed into red cells and to be added to the developing red cell mass in the lumen. The observations demonstrated in this figure in origin of red cells agree with Heitzman (1872) who believed that the protoplasm of hematoblastic substance can break into fragments which are themselves turned into red cells. H&E x 400

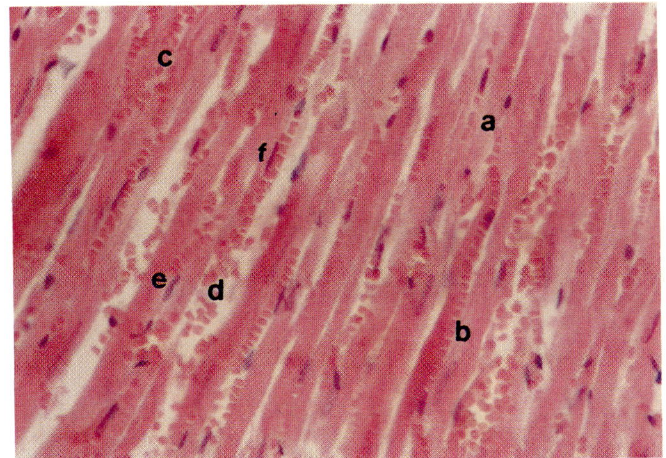

Figure 12

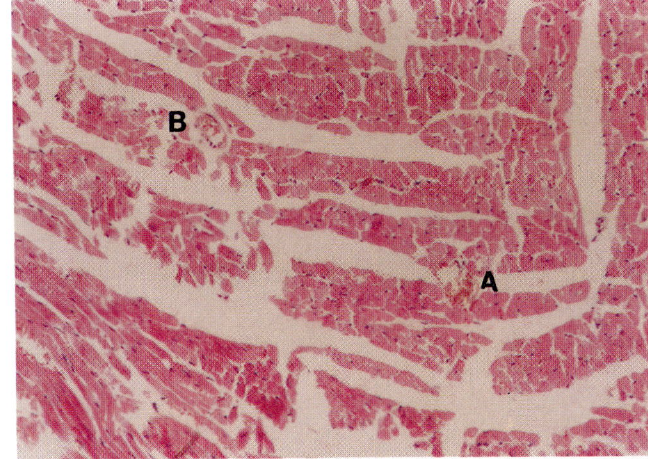

Figure 12-1

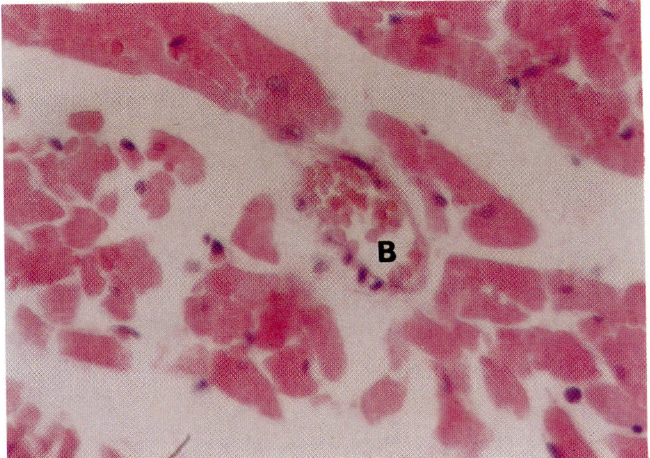

Figure 12-2

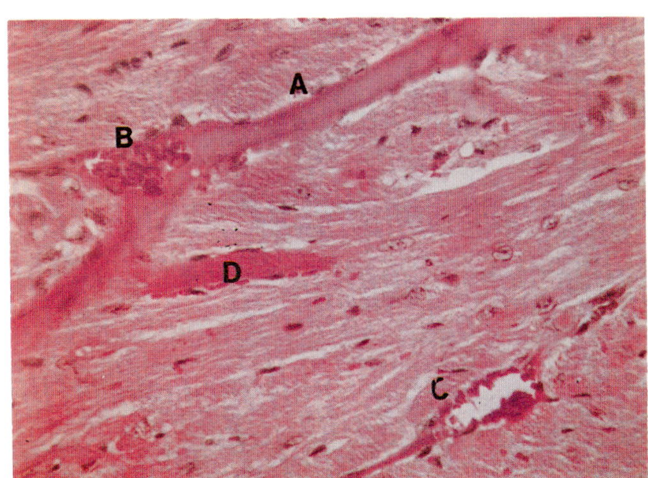

Figure 13

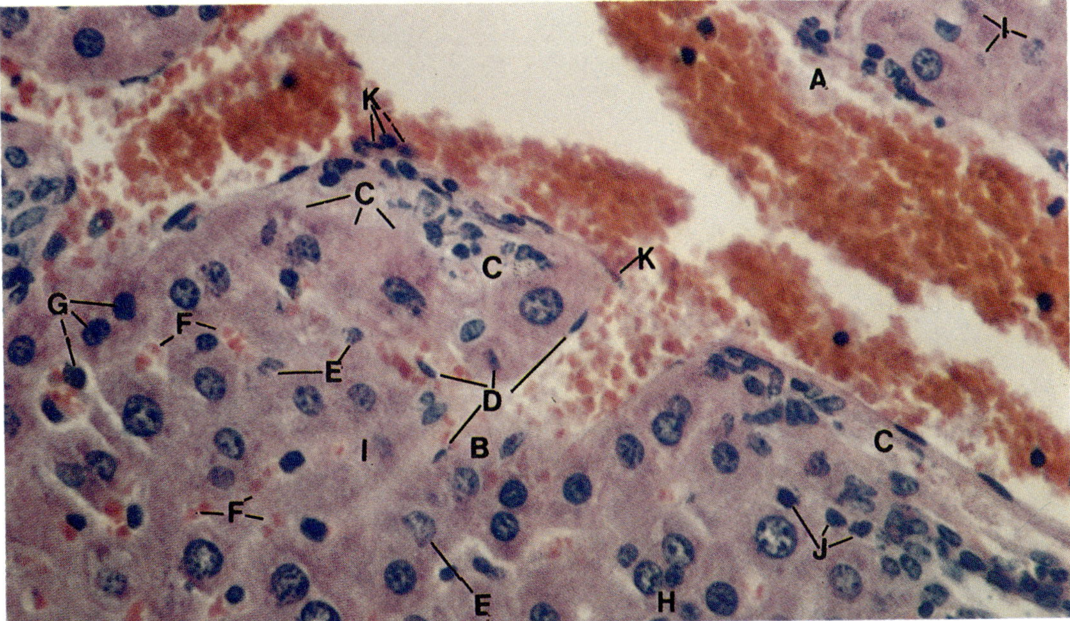

Figure 13-1

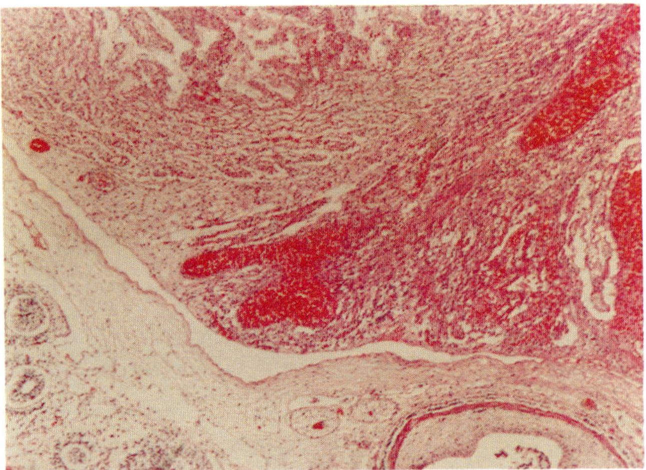

Figure 14

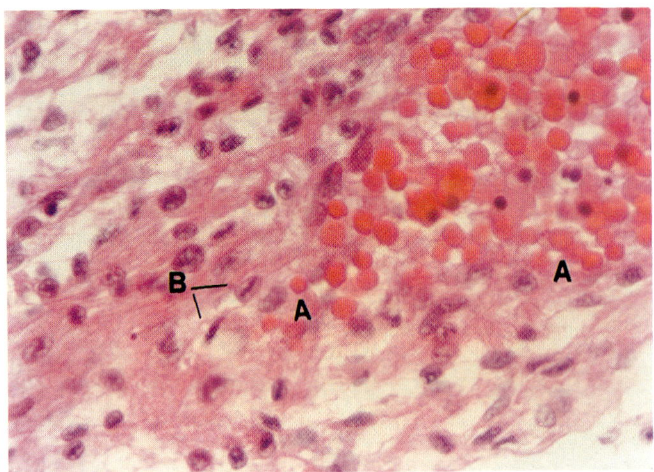

Figure 14-1

6. Embryological study of cardiac muscle (figs.14 to 15)

Embryonic cardiac muscle having the same capacity as adult cardiac muscle to form red cells directly, demonstrated in human embryo (figs. 14 and 14-1); and in chick embryo (fig. 15)

Figure 14 and 14-1. Upon casual observation of figure 14 one may designate the large amounts of blood occupying the mid and right areas of the field as a hemorrhage. With careful examination at a higher magnification (fig. 14-1) one can see that the myoplasm is transforming into red cells in areas (A). Note that in a few red cells there are tiny chromatin dot-like bodies known as Howell-Jolly bodies. Occasionally they are seen in blood smears from adults. It is interesting to note that occasionally cardiac muscle nuclei are taking the appearance of Anitschkow myocyte nuclei (B). Figure 14, H&E x 52; and figure 14-1, H&E x 520

Figure 15. In area (A), embryonic cardiac muscle cells are changing their nuclear characteristics to become small and lymphocyte-like. The cytoplasm is becoming orange in color and the shape of the cells is getting more spindle-shaped. In area (B), as in some other areas, red cells are becoming loose. The clear spaces, which represent plasma, are created by the dissolution of the muscle substance not involved in red cell formation. (C) points to an endothelial nucleus developing in the projected endothelial membrane surrounding the large island of developing red cells and plasma. H&E x 520

7. Chick embryonic cardiac muscle **in vitro** (figs. 16 to 16-3)

The possibility of development of red cells from 7-day-old chick embryonic cardiac muscle in vitro (figs. 16 and 16-1)
(In vitro growth of chick embryonic cardiac muscle for 4 days, fig. 16; and for 7 days fig. 16-1)

Figures 16 and 16-1. Note from the cultured muscle cells the origin of many small, round, possibly developing red cells with a tiny single nucleus (fig. 16). Further developmental stages with enlargement in size and possible increase in hemoglobin concentration are shown in figure16-1. At this stage these developing red cells are not showing any tendency to acquire spindle-shape, which is normal for chickens, both in adult and embryonic life (fig. 15). Figure 16, H&E x 520; and figure 16-1, H&E x 260

Capacity for intracellular development of fat by 12-day-old chick embryonic cardiac muscle in vitro (figs. 16-2 and 16-3)
(In vitro growth of chick embryonic cardiac muscle for 4 days, fig. 16-2; and for 8 days, fig. 16-3)

Figures 16-2 and 16-3. Both these photomicrographs reveal the development of fat in growing cardiac muscle *in vitro*. In figure 16-2 the fat appears as variable sizes of round vacuoles in H&E stain because the fat has been removed by alcohol and xylene during the normal staining process. Figure 16-3 shows the presence of small and large red globules representing fat stained by Oil O Red method. Figure 16-2, H&E x 400; and figure 16-3, Oil O Red x 325

fluid or the presence of what have been called large lymphatic channels in the myocardium without evidence of compression of peripheral muscle fibers should raise the question whether replacement of the muscle tissue by fluid may have occurred. This is exactly what is found by following the successive stages of development of these channels from cardiac muscle following lysis (figs. 35-37 and 38). Extensive lysis of cardiac muscle as presented here must have been the cause of cardiac failure in some patients with acute rheumatic fever. It may also be the cause of blockage in the conduction system, giving rise to different types of arrhythmias. The author has found that marked myocardial lysis without much evidence of reactive phenomenon is seen in many non-rheumatic-fever autopsy specimens, particularly in cases of carbon monoxide poisoning, diptheria, and in cases of violent death.

3. Hyalin degeneration

In the third type of degeneration, hyalin degeneration, the damaged muscle fibers have a ground-glass or wax-like appearance. The replacement of the regular muscle cell nuclei with large blotchy multinucleated vesicular forms is also a common characteristic of hyalin degeneration producing Type C Aschoff cells. This type of degeneration is most prominently seen in figures 28 and 28-1.

4. Fibrillary / fibrinoid degeneration

Prominent fibrillary/fibrinoid degeneration involving the inner myocardium with no attempts for Aschoff body formation is shown by figs. 49 and 50. It is possible that such occurrences could be followed by Aschoff body formation and fibrosis.

IV. REACTIVE PHENOMENON AND SUBSEQUENT DEVELOPMENT DEMONSTRATED BY DAMAGED MUSCLES

Damaged cardiac muscles typically exhibit several different types of reactive phenomena, according to the type of degeneration occurring. These include the formation of type specific Aschoff cells in production of Aschoff bodies which are the diagnostic feature of rheumatic fever. In some of these bodies there is evidence of abortive attempts or atypical regeneration of cardiac muscle. Following damage of the cardiac muscle, in addition to Aschoff body formation there may occur regeneration of normal cardiac muscle, formation of vascular channels, and fibrosis. Also, there may be an almost total absence of reactive phenomena in highly and acutely damaged muscle by lysis as shown in figure 36-1.

There are three particular components that may take part in the composition of Aschoff bodies: Aschoff cells; fibrinoid material; and a few non-specific cells such as lymphocytes, plasma cells, and occasionally a few other unspecified cells. The author's continued studies show that all these cells are derived from damaged cardiac muscle. According to different morphological characteristics Aschoff cells may be classified into three types (A, B and C) and their origin primarily follows three different pathways from cardiac muscle fibers having undergone three different types of degenerative processes, namely: 1. mixed degeneration; 2. cellular lysis; and 3. hyalin degeneration. These three types of Aschoff cells are designated by the author as Type A, Type B, and Type C Aschoff cells, respectively. The corresponding pathways of cytogenesis in the formation of these three different types of Aschoff cells from damaged cardiac muscle fibers are also termed by the author as Type A, B, and C (McDonald and Calkins, 1978). Aschoff bodies may contain more than one type of Aschoff cells. An Aschoff body containing primarily Types A and B Aschoff cells can be seen in figure 31. The Aschoff body in figure 29 contains all three types of cells with Type C being the most prominent.

1. Type 'A' cytogenesis in development of Type 'A' Aschoff cells through Anitschkow myocyte stages

Mixed degeneration—including fibrillary, fibrinoid, vacuolar, hyalin, and liquefaction degeneration—of myofibers may give rise to Anitschkow myocytes (an early stage of Type A Aschoff cells) through Type A cytogenesis (fig. 30). Here, the cardiac muscle cell nuclei may be transformed into that of Anitschkow myocytes. Anitschkow myocytes are described as having a narrow, central chromatin bar with a serrated margin and clear nucleoplasm. In a transverse section, these nuclei appear as a dark, central chromatin dot surrounded by clear nucleoplasm. (These cells are sometimes termed caterpillar cells. Compare figure 30 with figure 32; and figure 26 with figure 33.) The early investigators of Anitschkow's myocyte cells believed that they arose from cardiac muscle fibers. Oppel, who first described these cells in 1901, called them cells of muscle origin. In 1913 Anitschkow, while studying the formation of granulation tissue in the myocardium of rabbits, observed these cells. He coined the name "myocyte" since he traced the successive stages of their origin from the muscle fibers of the heart.

Individual cardiac muscle fibers from

which regular nuclei have already disappeared may also produce multiple Anitschkow myocytes without mitosis from changed myoplasm (fig. 31) in which striations are no longer present. Type A Aschoff cells, which represent a further developmental process of Anitschkow myocytes, exhibit irregular margins and reddish or bluish cytoplasm in H&E stain. They contain single or multiple nuclei and are commonly termed owl-eyed Aschoff cells (fig. 26). Similar observations, shown in figures 32 and 33, were made by Anitschkow in 1913. In rheumatic fever Anitschkow myocytes in large numbers may also be formed from the myogenic connective tissue of cardiac valves when acute inflammatory reaction with or without Aschoff body formation may be seen (figs. 52-54). The rare presence of Anitschkow myocytes originating within normal myofibers may be seen in non-rheumatic infant hearts (figs. 30-1 and 37-3).

2. Type 'B' cytogenesis in development of Type 'B' Aschoff cells from dedifferentiated tiny cells of muscle origin and followed by atypical muscle regeneration

Among many other important structural developments, cellular lysis leads to the formation of Type B Aschoff cells through Type B cytogenesis. Type B Aschoff cells are irregular, elongated, variable in size, and are characterized by ragged edges. The nuclei of these cells are usually hyperchromatic and show smudging (figs. 35, 36, 38-40, 42 and 43). Type B cytogenesis (McDonald 1957, 1975a, and McDonald and Calkins 1978) involves the appearance of tiny, hyperchromatic, round lymphocyte-like or tiny spindle-shaped nuclei within lysing cardiac muscle fibers, while the original muscle nuclei have already disappeared. These phenomena may be visualized by studying the sections of myocardium in figures 26 and 36. These tiny dedifferentiated nuclei with attached fibrils, derived from liquefied muscle product, may arrange themselves in a spindle pattern as the beginning of spindle-shaped Aschoff bodies. These dedifferentiated cells gradually accumulate shaggy, fibrinoid, irregular cytoplasm in their further development towards Type B Aschoff cells of

Aschoff bodies (figs. 38-40 and 42-45). The shaggy cytoplasm of these developing cells may turn into myoplasm with cross striations and with characteristic affinity for muscle stains. As mentioned earlier in this chapter, in the Aschoff body the degenerating myoplasm (figs. 26 and 27), as well as the regenerating myoplasm (figs. 40 and 42), may look like damaged collagen before the development of cross striations.

The myogenic origin of Aschoff bodies and the regeneration of cardiac muscle from Aschoff cells have been demonstrated with photomicrographs as early as 1920 by Whitman and Eastlake, and later by Murphy (1952 and 1959), McDonald (1957), McDonald (1975a), and McDonald and Calkins (1978). Aschoff body formation with Type B Aschoff cells may represent an abortive and atypical way of muscle regeneration which is peculiar to rheumatic fever. The development of muscle fibers from Aschoff cells within the Aschoff body takes place at a slower pace compared to the development of muscle fibers directly from the dedifferentiated cells outside the Aschoff bodies (figs. 40-42). This type of Aschoff body seems to be an atypical way of muscle formation in a nodular form (figs. 40 and 42-45).

3. Type 'C' cytogenesis in development of Type 'C' Aschoff cells

Finally, hyalin degeneration of individual muscle fibers is associated with the origin of Type C Aschoff cells through Type C cytogenesis. These cells usually contain large often multiple vesicular irregular nuclei with the replacement of regular cardiac muscle nuclei and light basophilic, waxy hyalinized cytoplasm. Type C Aschoff cells often resemble the Reed-Sternberg cells of Hodgkin's disease (figs. 28 and 29). Type C cytogenesis begins with hyalinization of cardiac muscle fibers at the central part of the cells while a rim of striated myoplasm may still be recognized at the periphery. This process subsequently results in the production of Type C Aschoff cells with the replacement of normal muscle fiber (fig. 45).

V. SUBSEQUENT DEVELOPMENT FOLLOWING LYSIS OF CARDIAC MUSCLE INCLUDING MYOCYTOLYSIS

In exceptionally acute fulminating cases of rheumatic fever with rapid myocardial lysis there may occur vary little reactive phenomena (as shown in fig. 36-1) with difficulty in making a histologically correct diagnosis. Usually even in fatal cases of acute rheumatic fever various reparative phenomena occur concurrently and side by side in the area of previous muscle lysis; these include: Aschoff body formation, regeneration of cardiac mus-

cle, fat infiltration, development of vascular channels, and development of collagenous fibrous tissue. Also rarely there may be almost the absence of reaction in acute fulminating rheumatic fever (fig. 36-1). Usually, more than one reparative phenomena can be seen side by side in the same section. For example, figure 40 shows a developing Aschoff body close to the area where normal regeneration of muscle (arrow) is occurring. Also in figures

37, 37-1 and 38 one can see vascular channels developing in the same general area in which Aschoff bodies are arising. All of these activities have started utilizing the original product of muscle lysis.

1. Regeneration of cardiac muscle and also possible intracellular fat production in outer myocardium following myocytolysis

In addition to the abortive and atypical way of muscle regeneration within Aschoff bodies described earlier, normal regeneration of cardiac muscle starting as similar tiny dedifferentiated cells occurs more imperceptibly outside Aschoff bodies. Instead of a mitotic basis for cell proliferation or maintenance of cell population, the lysing cardiac muscle cells give rise to multiple tiny, hyperchromatic cells in 'seed state', with or without discernable cytoplasm (figs. 35 and 36). These dedifferentiated cells in seed state possess remarkable potential to redifferentiate into normal striated muscle cells. The normal development of new muscle fibers from dedifferentiated cells may take place, often imperceptibly, along the margin and the interior of the cleft-like spaces of muscle lysis (figs. 40-42) thus narrowing the original tract of muscle lysis.

Lysis of individual cardiac muscle fibers in the subepicardial region (outer myocardium) usually leaves the sarcolemma more or less intact (myocytolysis). In such areas, the development of new muscle fibers may take place from dedifferentiated cells which are derived from lysing muscle cell products (fig. 47). The myoblast stages are usually demonstrable within the retained or newly formed sarcolemmal boundary (fig. 47). Without a stimulus for the regeneration of muscle, the content lined by remaining sarcolemma of individual muscle cells may be replaced with fatty substance and turned into adipose tissue. Compare figure 47 and 48 with figures 16-2 and 16-3 in which there is intracellular development of fat in cardiac muscle *in vitro*. Such a phenomenon was referred to by Coombs (1907, 1909, and 1924) who noted the infiltration of the muscle cells with fat in rheumatic fever.

Many investigators could not explain the increased number of muscle fibers which were observed in cardiac hypertrophy (increased muscle mass), since there is no suggestion of mitosis, mitotic division of nuclei, or splitting of myofibers. This detailed study showing the origin of cardiac muscle fibers from tiny dedifferentiated cells arising in lysing or liquefied muscle substance perhaps answers this query. The importance of these findings is the recognition of a direct attempt to repair the myocardial damage by regeneration of cardiac muscle. A similar observation was made by Spiedel (1938) in his experiment with living skeletal muscle when he noted tiny dedifferentiated cells arose in skeletal muscle and formed new muscle fibers. Similar dedifferentiated cells are described by Mauro (1961) and Church, Noronha, and Allbrook (1966) as satellite cells having a remarkable potential for regeneration of skeletal muscle in case of injury. These satellite cells are similar to dedifferentiated cells, mostly lymphocyte-like bare nuclei, and usually arise at the periphery of the damaged muscle fibers. In the absence of stimulation for muscle regeneration, these dedifferentiated cells, as well as Anitschkow myocytes, take part in the creation of fibrous tissue which may fill the remaining gaps created by muscle lysis (figs. 25 and 46). This process will be discussed in detail below.

2. Development of vascular channels from the product of muscle lysis

Another development from cardiac muscle which has undergone cellular lysis is the formation of vascular channels. During the process of repair of myocardial lysis, endothelial membranes enclosing the columns of liquid may develop probably as a protective mechanism from further lysis of peripheral myofibers (figs. 34, 36-1, 37 and 38), and such channels become known as lymphatic channels. The development of lymphatic channels following cellular lysis is not limited only to rheumatic fever. In fact, this is the natural way of vessel formation. Also red cells may develop from lysing muscle fibers and contribute to the development of blood vessels (fig. 37-2). (The development of blood and blood vessels from cardiac muscle fibers is demonstrated in great detail in chapter one of this volume.)

3. Frequent association of Aschoff bodies with vascular channels

In addition to the misconception that Aschoff bodies arise from interstitial collagenous tissue of myocardium, there is another less known supposition stating that Aschoff bodies arise from the perivascular connective tissue. The latter supposition might have been developed from casual observations of histological structures as shown in figure 37-1, not taking into account that a long track of muscle has been replaced in development of this vessel and the surrounding Aschoff bodies and the loose connective tissue. After examining the developmental processes in figures 35 to 38, one can easily see the reason for close association of Aschoff bodies and vascular channels. In fact, these two structures actually demonstrate two different reactive phenomena occurring in the same area of muscle lysis. Soon the endothelial membrane retracts from the peripheral surviving muscle and the gap gets filled up by regenerating cardiac muscle and/or the collageneous connective tissue with or without Aschoff body formation as shown in figure 37-1.

4. Development of collageneous fibrous tissue from damaged cardiac muscle

As mentioned at the beginning of this chapter, the current theory hypothesizes that the Aschoff body is derived from collagenous tissue rather than from the cardiac muscle itself. Indeed, Aschoff bodies can be frequently seen in association with fibrous tissue in the myocardium (see figures 25 and 46); however, as demonstrated, these bands of fibrous tissue do not produce Aschoff bodies, but rather the fibrous tissue itself originates in the tracts derived from previous cell lysis, and signifies a lack of stimulus for the full amount of muscle regeneration. Therefore, in addition to the regenerating muscle fibers shown in Aschoff bodies and in the area of previous cellular lysis (figs. 40-42), a small amount of collagenous fibers may develop in association with dedifferentiated cells or from Anitschkow myocytes. These findings suggest the potential of myogenic cells to redifferentiate into fibrous connective cells and also that such an occurrence is responsible for the fibrous scarring of myocardium as shown in chronic (fig. 25) and also the earlier stages (fig. 46) of rheumatic fever.

Fibrous thickening of the endocardium may be initiated by extensive fibrillary/fibrinoid degeneration of subendocardial cardiac muscle (figs. 49-50). Aschoff bodies may also be present in this region (figs. 23 and 26) a long time after the acute condition has subsided.

5. Possible absence of reactive phenomena following extensive and rapid myocardial lysis in acute fulminating rheumatic fever

In rare cases of acute rheumatic fever, the injurious effect may be so overwhelming that there may not be any detectable attempt for repair following extensive lysis of muscle tissue. In these rare cases, all of the clinical symptoms of rheumatic fever are present, but the diagnosis is difficult to confirm histologically because of the difficulty encountered in finding an Aschoff body in the cardiac muscle. Some of these cases may go undiagnosed. This phenomenon is shown in figure 36-1 where evidence for only a small reaction—the development of delicate capillaries from the lysing muscle product—can actually be seen.

VI. AUTHOR'S COMMENTS AND EXPLANATION FOR THE MISCONCEPTION THAT COLLAGEN DEGENERATION IS THE PRIMARY DAMAGE IN RHEUMATIC FEVER

From this study it became clear that the damage of cardiac muscle itself is the main onslaught of acute rheumatic fever. Also, the origin of Aschoff bodies, the diagnostic feature of this disease, is derived from the damaged cardiac muscle tissue. The various cellular structures and the acellular fibrinoid material composing Aschoff bodies are found to be of myogenic origin. Anitschkow myocytes, which are one of the cellular components of Aschoff bodies and other Aschoff cells, thought to be derived from connective tissue, are actually found to be of myogenic origin (McDonald 1957, 1963a, 1975a, and McDonald and Calkins 1978). Aschoff (1939) stated in his article, "It is in no way essential that the formation of the richly cellular nodules should be preceded by fibrinoid degeneration of ground substance." One must remember that there is hardly any collagenous fibrous tissue in the normal healthy myocardium of children. It is no wonder that so many children have died of acute cardiac failure as a result of extensive myocadial damage, particularly by dissolution of cardiac muscle.

Because rheumatic fever is commonly considered a collagen disease, the damage of cardiac muscle and its various reactive changes have been ignored. Gould (1960 p. 660) stated, "The discrepancy so frequently observed between the degree of functional impairment and the minor morphological signs of inflammation (Aschoff bodies) demonstrable by the pathologists has led many to postulate and search for evidence of direct injury to the myocardial fibers." He also stated, "The inadequacy of histologic methods to demonstrate such changes so deplored by Coombs (1907, 1909 and 1924) many years ago, still remains." The author's demonstrations of the extensive damage of cardiac muscle in acute rheumatic fever in this volume and in earlier publications (McDonald 1957, 1963ab 1975a and McDonald and Calkins, 1978), refute the inadequacy of histologic methods. In fact, simple histologic technique is a great tool to view a whole spectrum of life cycles of cells and tissues. In tissue sections one can see in relatively unaltered forms the cross sections of various morphological activities proceeding in time.

The theory that rheumatic fever is a collagen disease was probably developed for several reasons. This theory is based mainly on the presence of what is perceived to be, on casual observation, degenerated collagen in the Aschoff body. This 'degenerated collagen' is shown by the author to be an acellular degenerated fibrin-like material which is actually found to be of muscle origin. The author, in agreement with the findings of Whitman and Eastlake (1920) and Murphy (1952 and 1959) believes that degenerating as well as regenerating myoplasm, before the development of cross striations, has the appearance of damaged collagen. In chronic and subacute cases one often sees Aschoff bodies in association with developing fibrous collagenous tissue derived from imperfect healing process. This fact may also be partly responsible for the deduction that Aschoff bodies arise from collagenous tissue (figures 25 and 46) even though there are hardly any collagen fibers to begin with in the myocardium of a child. The author has shown that the collagen fibers are the product of an imperfect healing process of damaged muscle rather than the primary tissue for the origin of Aschoff bodies. Aschoff (1939) said in his last article, "It is in no way essential that the formation of the richly cellular nodules should be preceded by fibrinoid degeneration of ground substance." Another reason that acute rheumatic fever has been mistaken for a collagenous disease is that Anitschkow myocytes can be seen in collagenous tissue of the cardiac valves. The author explains this phenomenon by pointing out that cardiac valves, which are later formed of mainly collagenous tissue, are derived embryologically from cardiac muscle (figs. 22-1 and 22-2); so the fibrous tissue of valves have the same capacity as cardiac muscle in production of Anitschkow myocytes (see chapter two and figure 54).

The preconceived idea that rheumatic fever is a collagenous disease is mostly responsible for the general neglect in viewing the actual changes in cardiac muscle fibers. In acute cases, the clinical picture of cardiac failure is much more compatible with cardiac muscle damage than with collagen disease. In conclusion, it became clear through detailed histologic study of the myocardium of patients who died of acute rheumatic fever that the damage to cardiac muscle itself is the main onslaught of acute rheumatic fever.

VII. ACUTE INFLAMMATORY REACTION IN CARDIAC VALVES

In acute rheumatic fever, acute inflammatory reaction involving papillary muscle (fig. 51) and cardiac valve cusps (figs. 52-54) is commonly seen. Anitschkow myocytes play an important role in the production of inflammatory cells with peculiar morphology. The development of such atypical cellular structures from Anitschkow myocytes was demonstrated earlier (McDonald 1963)a. Occasionally, Aschoff body-like structures may develop in this area together with a dense proliferation of acute inflammatory cells. In chronic cases of rheumatic fever, focal damage of myocardium beneath the thickened endocardium along with the presence of Aschoff bodies signifies a delayed healing process (figs. 23-24) and causes further thickening of the endocardium. It is important to notice that many small cells derived from altered muscle fibers or from fibrous tissue of muscle origin fall under the categories of chronic or acute inflammatory cells such as lymphocytes, histiocytes, monocytes, plasma cells (infrequently), and in some locations, acute inflammatory cells (SN cells) with atypical configurations (figs. 52-53), (McDonald 1963a). In addition to Anitschkow myocytes taking part in the regeneration of cardiac muscles (fig. 44) and the development of fibrous tissue, they may take an active part in the development of these inflammatory cells (fig. 51). Figure 53 shows acute inflammatory cells arising from Anitschkow myocytes.

Without going into too much detail, figure 55 is included at the end of the chapter to show briefly the microscopic appearance of fibrinous pericarditis which occurs occasionally in acute rheumatic fever.

VIII. SUMMARY OF AUTHOR'S OBSERVATIONS PRESENTED IN THIS CHAPTER

The damage of cardiac muscle is found to be the main lesion and the possible cause of death in acute rheumatic fever. The development of Aschoff bodies, the diagnostic feature of rheumatic fever, starts with the damage (degeneration) of cardiac muscle. There are three different pathways (Types A, B and C) for the cytogenesis of corresponding types of Aschoff cells (A, B and C) from altered muscle fibers. The descriptive classification of myocardial Aschoff bodies as formulated by Gross and Ehrlich (1934) is found to be related to the types of cytogenesis and the various stages of Aschoff body development from damaged muscle. These classifications are also related to the regression of Aschoff bodies and also the regeneration of cardiac muscle fibers from Aschoff cells.

The cytogenesis of Type A Aschoff cells starting as Anitschkow myocytes from degenerated cardiac muscle cells is presented in figures 26 and 30-33, and their participation in formation of an Aschoff body in figures 26 and 31.

Type B cytogenesis, which starts with the lysis of cardiac muscle and is followed by the progressive development of tiny dedifferentiated cells arising from cardiac muscle that has undergone lysis, is seen in figures 27 and 45, and the development of Aschoff body in figure 27.

Type C cytogenesis starts with central hyalinization of muscle fibers followed by the development of Aschoff cells, with single or multiple large vesicular nuclei; the development of an Aschoff body is seen in figures 28, 28-1, 29 and 31 (C).

The development of an Aschoff body frequently involves a combination of different cytogenesis processes in the development of Aschoff cells. In addition, there are nonspecific cellular elements, some of which may be categorized as inflammatory cells of local origin as shown in figure 29. Damaged muscle element as well as regenerating muscle element following cellular lysis in Type B cytogenesis appear to be what is mistakenly known as fibrinoid degeneration of collagen.

Occasionally, the development of Anitschkow myocytes from cardiac muscles may be seen in non-rheumatic patients (figs. 30-1 and 37-3).

The developmental processes of fibrous thickening of endocardium from fibrillary-fibrinoid degeneration of cardiac muscle can be seen in figures 49 and 50. The development of fibrous scar in the myocardium (figs. 25 and 46) is due to insufficient muscle regeneration and fibrous tissue transformation of liquefied muscle with dedifferentiated

nuclei (figs. 36, 40 and 41).

The following morphological changes represent normal histological structures that may develop from the product of cell lysis: the regeneration of normal muscle fibers from dedifferentiated cells arising from lysing muscle in the lumen and at the edges of the clefts bordering surviving muscle bundles; the frequent development of endothelial-like membrane bordering the clefts filled with clear fluid of muscle lysis (commonly known as lymphatic channels); in the production of blood vessels, the possibility of red cell development from liquefied muscle product within the clefts lined by endothelium; and the development of collagenous fibrous scar tissue from liquefied muscle product due to incomplete muscle regeneration. Rarely there may be massive cellular lysis with no evidence of Aschoff body formation under overwhelming injurious effects of rheumatic fever (fig. 36-1).

Also explained in this study is how the Aschoff bodies of cardiac muscle origin acquire their perivascular position (figs. 37, 37-1 and 38) in the inner myocardium.

Lysis of intracellular sarcoplasm with retention of sarcolemma (myocytolysis) is usually seen in subepicardial myocardium. Regeneration of cardiac muscle fibers within retained or newly formed sarcolemma and the possibility of Aschoff body formation following myocytolysis are shown in figures 47 and 48 respectively. Another reaction in acute rheumatic fever is the proliferation of acute inflammatory cells in cardiac valves and in subendocardial cardiac muscle, including that of the papillary muscle (figs. 51-53).

IX. EXPLANATION OF FIGURES AND CASE HISTORIES

Of the 59 photomicrographs in this chapter, 21 have been reproduced in color from previously published articles: figures 26, 30, and 31 are from McDonald (1963a); figures 34-36, 38-43, 47 and 48 are from McDonald (1975a); and figures 28, 28-1, 29, 44, 45, 49 and 50 are from McDonald and Calkins (1978). These pictures have been reproduced with the permission of their publishers.

All figures (23-55) shown in this chapter are taken from the postmortem specimens of the left ventricular myocardium of eight patients who died of acute rheumatic fever with the following exceptions: figures 23 and 24, surgical specimens of atrial appendage from two patients with chronic rheumatic fever. The patient of figure 24 died on the thirteenth post-commissurotomy day. The autopsy specimen of the left ventricular myocardium of this patient is also included (fig. 25). Figures 32 and 33 are photographic reproduc

tions of hand-drawn pictures of Anitschkow myocyte development by Anitschkow (1913); and figures 30-1 and 37-3, autopsy specimens of left ventricular myocardium of two non-rheumatic infants. Figure 51 is from papillary muscle; figures 52-54 from mitral valve cusps; and figure 55 is from the visceral pericardium.

Case No. 1, (fig. 23): A 30-year-old patient with a past history of chronic rheumatic fever suffering from mitral stenosis with congestive failure. Surgical specimen of atrial appendage of heart was removed by mitral commissurotomy.

Case No. 2, (figs. 24 and 25): A 27-year-old male with a past history of chronic rheumatic heart disease underwent mitral commissurotomy for the treatment of mitral stenosis. The patient died 13 days later. This patient showed no clinical signs of rheumatic activity. Figure 24 is a surgical specimen from the atrial appendage. Figure 25 is from the autopsy specimen of the left ventricular myocardium.

Case No. 3, (figs. 26, 30, 44 and 45): A 9-year-old boy who was admitted with a two-month history of intermittent joint pain and precordial pain for eight days. He developed mild decompensation and died seven weeks after hospital admission. At autopsy, the heart muscle was flabby and the chambers were dilated. Fine verrucci were present in the line of closure of the aortic and mitral valves.

Case No. 4, (figs. 27, 35, 36, 37, 38-43 and 46) ventricular myocardium; (fig. 51) papillary muscle; and (figs. 52-54) mitral valve cusp: A 17-year-old girl who was admitted because of swollen ankle joints, fever for two weeks, and anemia. She died on the fourth day in the hospital with a diagnosis of acute rheumatic fever. The mitral valve was thickened and showed a row of slightly elevated nodules along the free margin.

Case No. 5, (figs. 28, 28-1, 29 and 31): A 4-year-old girl who was admitted with fever, swollen and tender joints, and ankle edema. Acute rheumatic heart disease was diagnosed. The child went home after an eight week stay in the hospital but returned with acute cardiac failure and died after three weeks.

Case No. 6, (figs. 34 and 47): A 9-year-old boy who developed joint symptoms followed by cardiac ailments and died eighteen months later of acute rheumatic heart disease. At autopsy the heart weighed 280 gms. Fibrinous exudate was noticed over the pericardium. The myocardium was soft and flabby and verrucci were present at the free edges of the cardiac valves.

Case No. 7, (fig. 36-1): A 22-year-old male who was admitted with the diagnosis of acute fulminating rheumatic heart disease and died shortly thereafter. The clinical diagnosis was mitral insufficiency, endocarditis, and cardiac dilatation with marked fatty degeneration of the heart muscle.

Case No. 8, (figs. 37-2 and 48-50): An 11-year-old boy who was admitted and was diagnosed as having acute rheumatic heart disease with congestive heart failure. The first onset of joint symptoms was four months before this admission. He died ten months after his admission. At autopsy the heart weighed 500 gms. The epicardial surface was roughened and lined with fibrinous exudate. The mitral valve was thickened and sand-like nodules were noticed at the line of closure of the cardiac valves.

Case No. 9, (fig. 55) visceral pericardium: A 9-year-old boy with a history of frequent sore throats and shifting joint pain, he died of acute rheumatic heart disease on the sixth day after hospital admission. The postmortem diagnosis included acute rheumatic myocarditis, endocarditis, and fibrinous pericarditis.

Case No. 10, (fig. 37-1): An autopsy specimen of the myocardium of a patient with acute rheumatic fever (further history not available).

Cases No. 11 and 12 are cardiac muscle from two non-rheumatic patients. Case No. 11, (fig. 30-1): A 22-month-old boy who died of bronchopneumonia. Case No. 12, (fig. 37-3): A 3-week-old boy who died of a congenital heart defect.

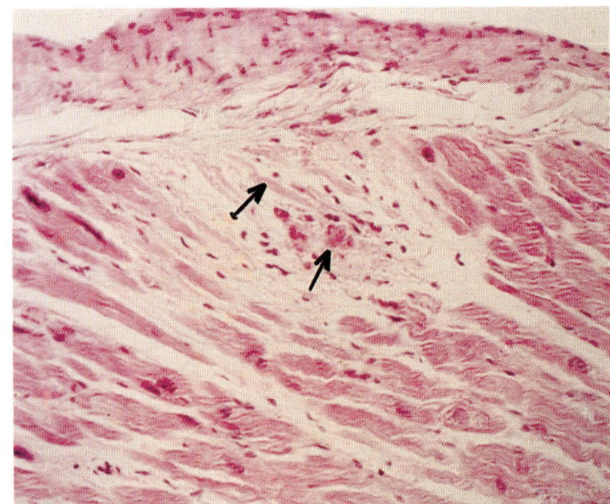

Figure 23

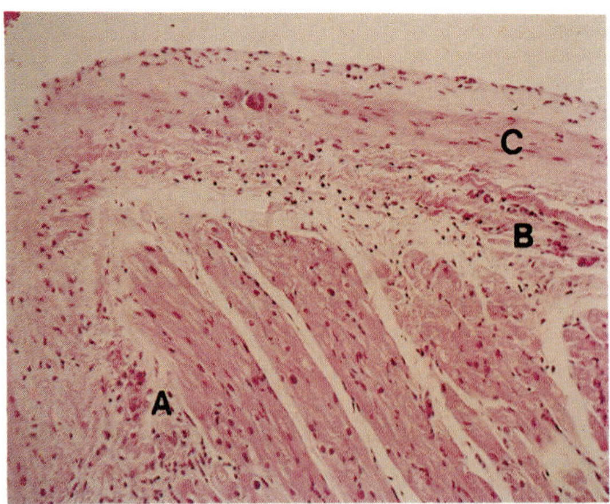

Figure 24

1. The development of thickened endocardium caused by rheumatic fever lesions with Aschoff body formation (figs. 23 and 24)

Figure 23. Focal damage of cardiac muscle in the subendocardial region with production of fibrinoid material (arrows), and development of an Aschoff body is shown. H&E x 145

Figure 24. Continued rheumatic activity is reflected by the damaged cardiac muscle and the presence of an Aschoff body (A) together with other small, non-specific inflammatory cellular elements including a few SN cells. The Aschoff body (B) is separated from the cardiac muscle bundles below. The presence of smooth muscle (C) commonly seen in thickened endocardium replaces the original cardiac muscle (see figures 49 and 50 for the developing processes of thickened endocardium from extensively damaged cardiac muscle without much inflammatory reaction). H&E x 85

2. Chronic rheumatic disease process with the replacement of cardiac muscle by developing scar tissue (fig. 25)

Figure 25. The autopsy specimen (thirteenth post-commissurotomy day) of the left ventricular myocardium of the same patient as shown in figure 24 is presented here. This figure represents continued rheumatic activity and replacement of the damaged muscle with prominent linear fibrous scarring in which Aschoff bodies can still be recognized (arrow). There should be very little fibrous tissue in the myocardium of a normal 27-year-old person. H&E x 40

3. Cytogenesis of Aschoff bodies and Aschoff cells (figs. 26-42)

Degenerated muscle element giving rise to fibrinoid material and various types of Aschoff bodies (figs. 26-29); predominantly Type A Aschoff cells (fig. 26); Type B Aschoff cells (fig. 27); Type C Aschoff cells (figs. 28 & 28-1); the cytogenesis processes of Type C Aschoff cells from muscle fibers (figs. 28 and 28-1); mixtures of Types A, B and C Aschoff cells (fig. 29)

Figure 26. This figure illustrates mixed degenerative changes (including hyalin, fibrinoid/fibrillary degeneration and liquefaction) in cardiac muscle and the predominant appearance of Anitschkow myocytes and their further development into Type A, owl-eyed Aschoff cells with single, double or multiple nuclei (A). Note that many nuclei are presented in longitudinal as well as transverse planes of Anitschkow myocytes within the large multi-nucleated Aschoff cell. (See figures 30-33 for the progressive developmental stages of Anitschkow myocytes from cardiac muscle fiber.) (B) denotes earlier stages of Anitschkow myocytes in transverse planes as compared to what are indicated by (A). H&E x 800

Figure 27. Shown here is a spindle-shaped Aschoff body with Type B Aschoff cells having shaggy fibrillary eosinophilic cytoplasm and hyperchromatic nuclei of variable sizes. (A) points to a regenerating muscle fiber with partly fibrinoid cytoplasm derived through Type B cytogenesis (figures 35-45 demonstrate such cytogenesis processes). Appropriate staining methods have also shown that in addition to muscle regeneration a small amount of fibrillary material with or without being attached to the dedifferentiated nuclei acquires the affinity for collagen stains. H&E x 150

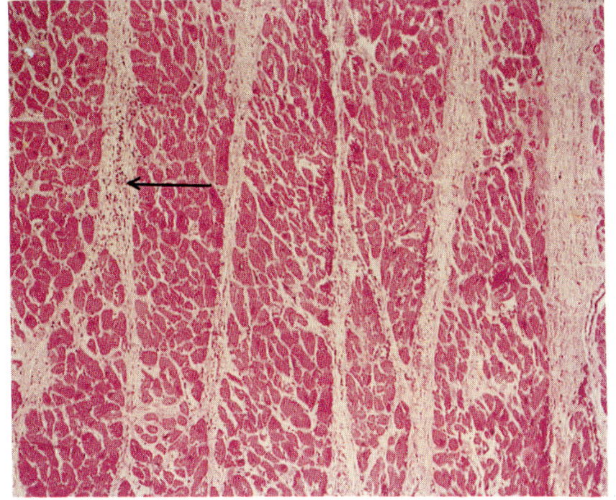

Figure 25

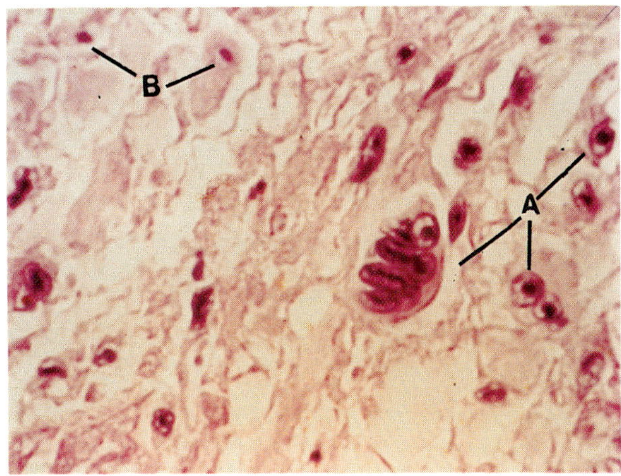

Figure 26

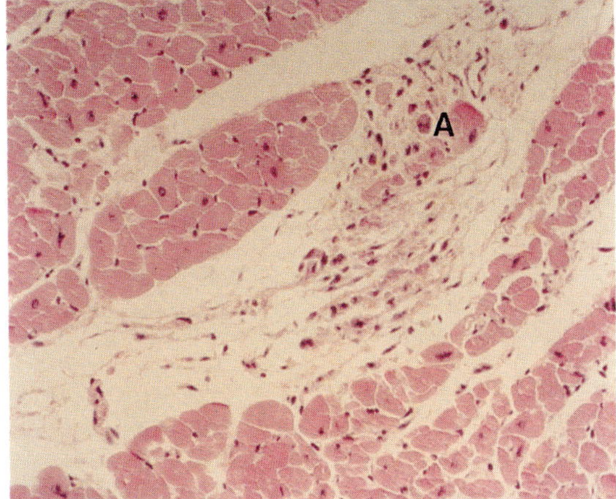

Figure 27

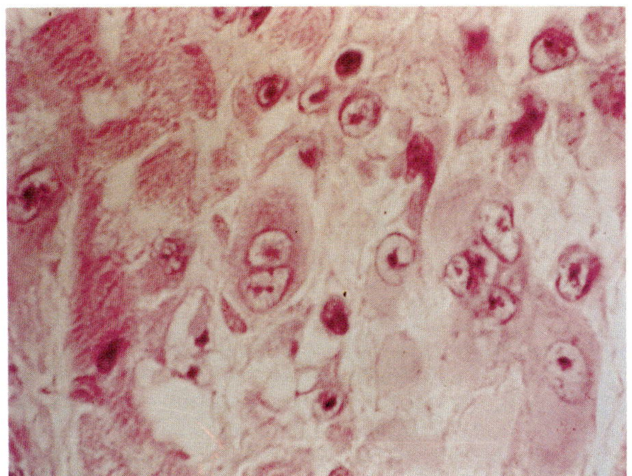

Figure 28

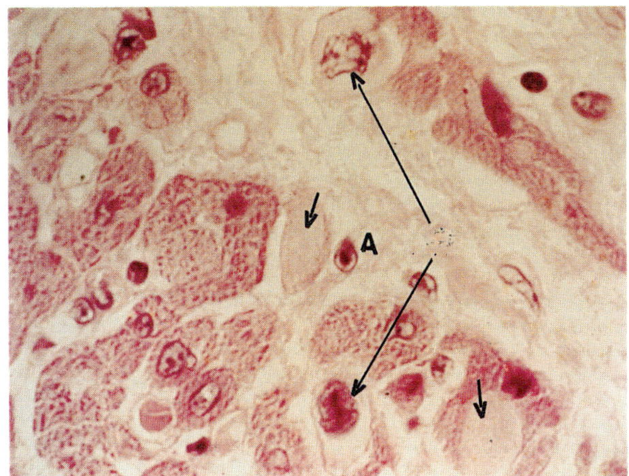

Figure 28-1

Figure 28. Presented here is a preponderance of Type C Aschoff cells with large, hyalinized, usually lightly basophilic cytoplasm and single or multiple large vesicular nuclei. The origin of such Aschoff cells associated with hyalinization is also shown in figures 28-1 and 31. H&E x 708

Figure 28-1. Shown here are Anitschkow myocytes (A) in a transverse plane. Within the cardiac muscle fibers Type C Aschoff cells appear (long arrows). The short arrows point to the hyalinized cytoplasm of developing Type C Aschoff cells, the nuclei of which are not in the planes of view. H&E x 708

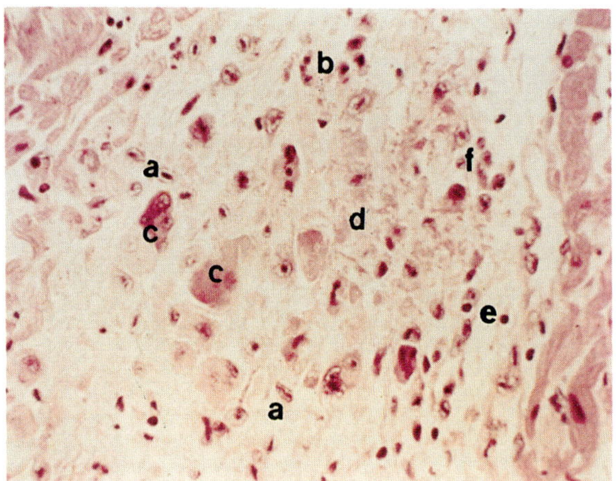

Figure 29

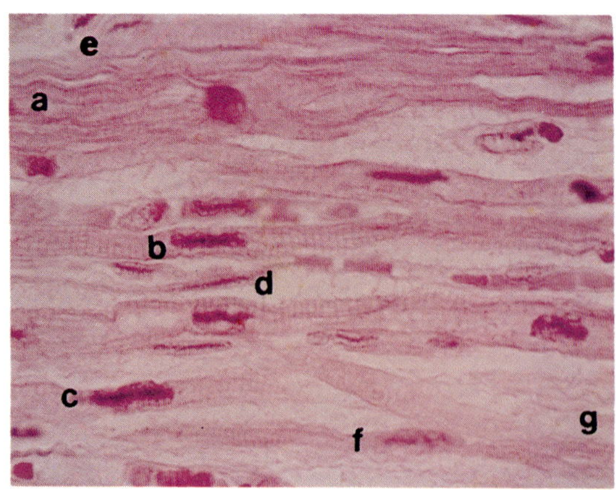

Figure 30

Figure 29. This figure demonstrates the polymorphic nature of the Aschoff body with different kinds of Aschoff cells arising from damaged muscle elements undergoing fibrinoid, hyalin, and liquefaction degeneration. Many Type A cells originate as Anitschkow myocytes (a) in longitudinal, oblique, and transverse planes. Tiny dedifferentiated nuclei (b) present an early stage of Type B Aschoff cell formation (see also figures 26 (B), 35 and 36). Several Type C Aschoff cells (c) have large hyalinized basophilic cytoplasm and single or multiple large, irregular nuclei. (The origin of such Aschoff cells directly from cardiac muscle fibers is better shown in figures 28 and 31.) Fibrinoid material (d), is usually misinterpreted as fibrinoid degeneration of collagen instead of fibrinoid degeneration of muscle. Several scattered tiny cells, a few of which may be classified as lymphocytes (e), and several other tiny nuclei resembling atypical Anitschkow myocytes (f) are shown; see also figure 31 (A). H&E x 292

Origin and multiplication of Anitschkow myocytes from cardiac muscle fibers (figs. 30-33)
(Figures 32 and 33 are reproductions of hand drawn figures by Anitschkow in 1913)

Figure 30. Successive stages of nuclear and sarcoplasmic changes in muscle fibers involving the development of Anitschkow myocytes (a-d) are depicted in this figure. Degeneration or alteration of muscle fibers seems to be associated with the origin of Anitschkow myocytes. The presence of the remaining myofibrils at both ends of the formative Anitschkow myocyte (d) appears to be responsible for keeping the long narrow shape of this nucleus. With dissolution of remaining myofibrils, the Anitschkow myocytes assume an oval form (e). Proliferation of Anitschkow myocytes as if by fragmentation within the

muscle fiber is shown by (f). Compare (f) with (A) in figure 31 for further evidence of multiple Anitschkow myocytes arising from a single muscle fiber without mitosis. (g) points to wavy fibrillary changes in muscle fibers, with the loss of cross striations. H&E x 500

Rarely non-rheumatic cardiac muscles may produce Anitschkow myocytes (fig. 30-1, see also fig. 37-3)

Figure 30-1. In a non-rheumatic heart, this figure shows an abrupt development of Anitschkow myocytes (A) from a cardiac muscle fiber in which the original shape of the muscle fiber and the cross striations are well retained. Note the origin of two Anitschkow myocytes (B) from a single muscle fiber; also note the transverse striations of myofibers that can still be seen within the developing Anitschkow myocyte (A). H&E x 1300

Figure 31. In this figure, Anitschkow myocyte nuclei are proliferating, in a large number, in a partly hyalinized and vacuolated cardiac muscle fiber (A). In the area of degenerated muscle fibers tiny scattered nuclei (B), representing the early stage of Type B Aschoff cells, with a small amount of ill-defined cytoplasm appear. (C) points to Type C Aschoff cells developing from a myofiber. H&E x 510

Figures 32 and 33. Reference is made here to the myogenic origin of Anitschkow myocytes as observed by Anitschkow (1913) while studying granulation tissue formation in rabbit myocardium. Reproductions of his hand-drawn figures depict successive cellular changes in cardiac muscle fibers in both longitudinal and transverse planes, with original number 19 for the present figure 32 and original numbers 23 and 24 for the present figure 33. Similar development of Anitschkow myocytes from cardiac muscle fibers is shown by the author in figures 26 and 30.

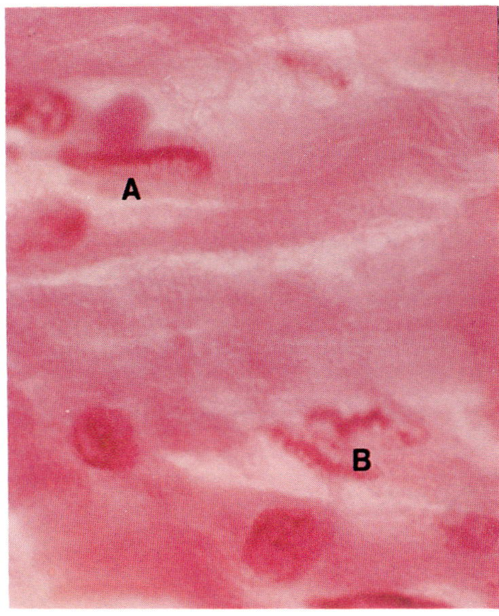

Figure 30-1

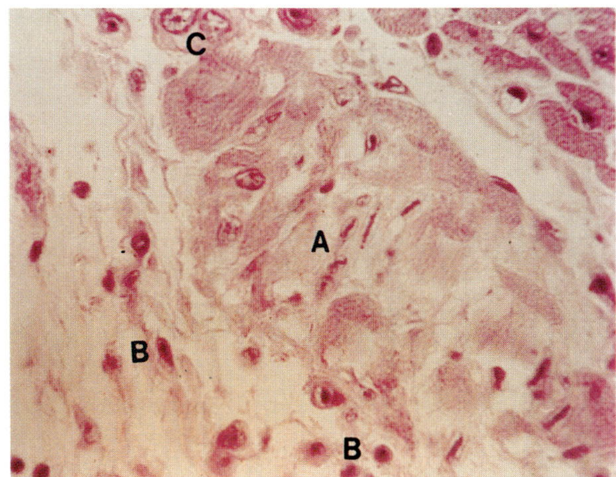

Figure 31

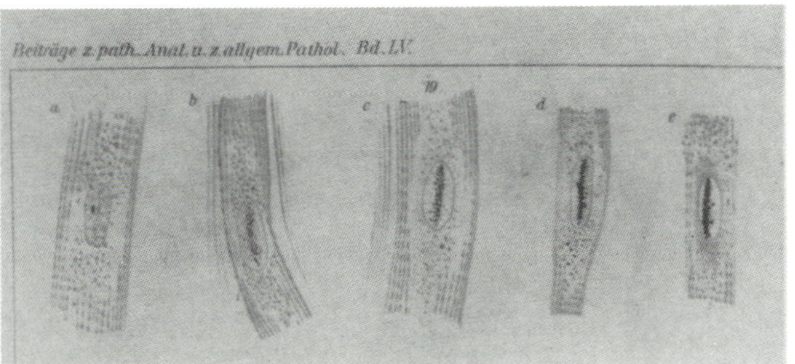

Figure 32

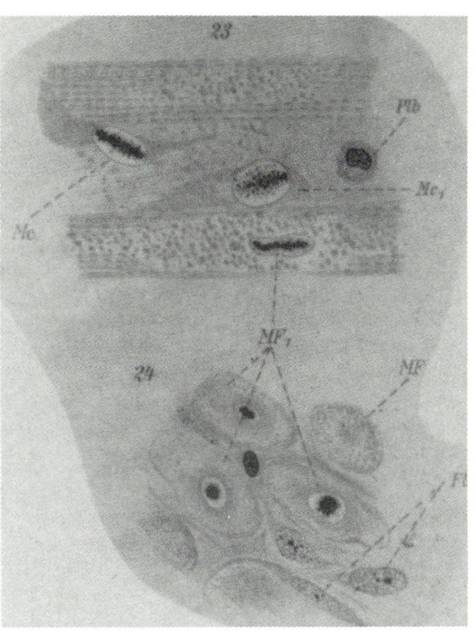

Figure 33

From liquefied muscle product—origin of tiny dedifferentiated cells with the capacity for Aschoff body formation with Type B Aschoff cells (figs. 34, 35, 36 and 38-42) and for regeneration of cardiac muscle within and outside Aschoff bodies (figs. 40-42); development of vascular channels (figs. 36-1 to 37-1) with blood formation (figs. 37-2 and 37-3)

Figure 34. Note the two wide clefts enclosing the clear fluid produced by myocardial lysis (also see figures 35 and 36). The upper cleft shows two developing vascular channels (commonly categorized as lymphatic channels) partially lined by a fine, delicate endothelial structure (arrows). A spindle-shaped Aschoff body (A) occupies a part of the lower cleft towards the right. (In the surrounding muscle there is a fine network of clear spaces formed by muscle lysis. Normally cardiac muscle fibers should be very compact.) H&E x 55

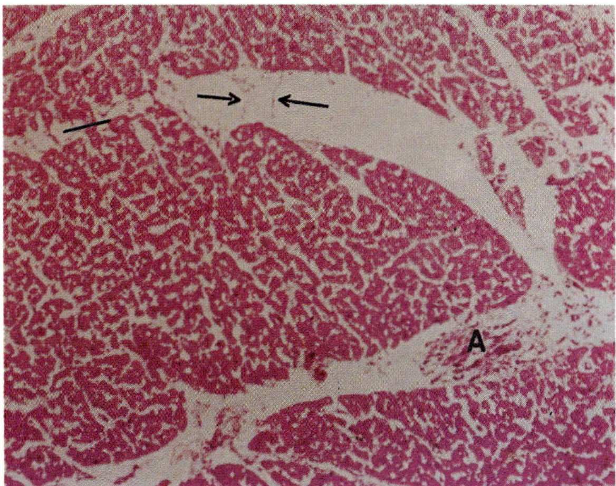

Figure 34

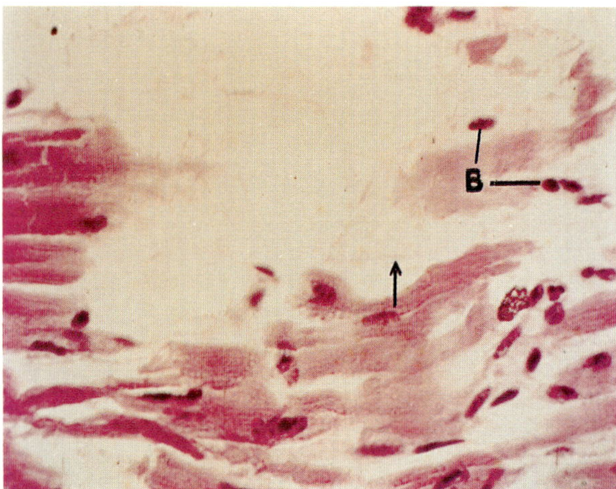

Figure 35

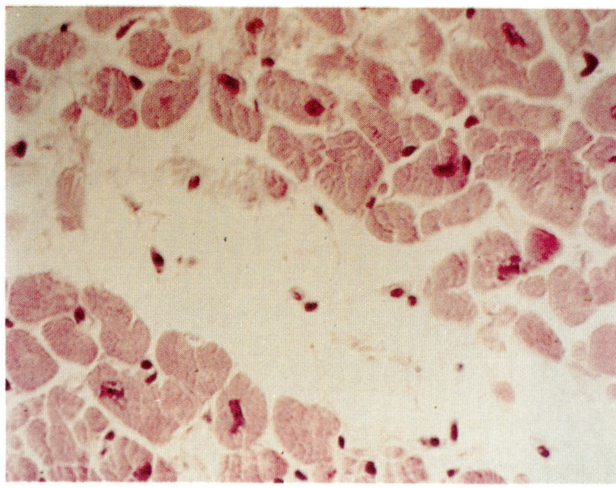

Figure 36

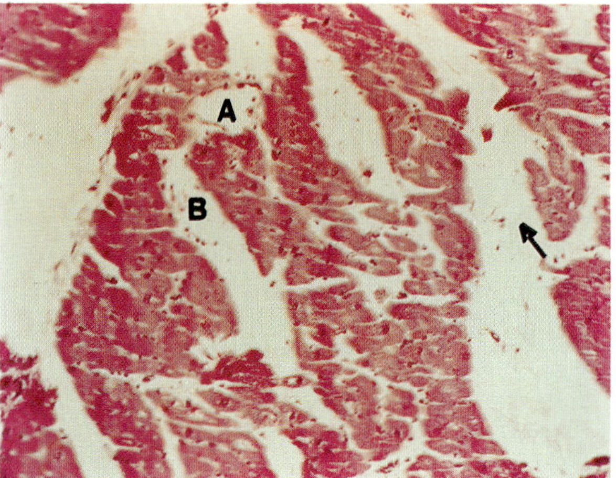

Figure 36-1

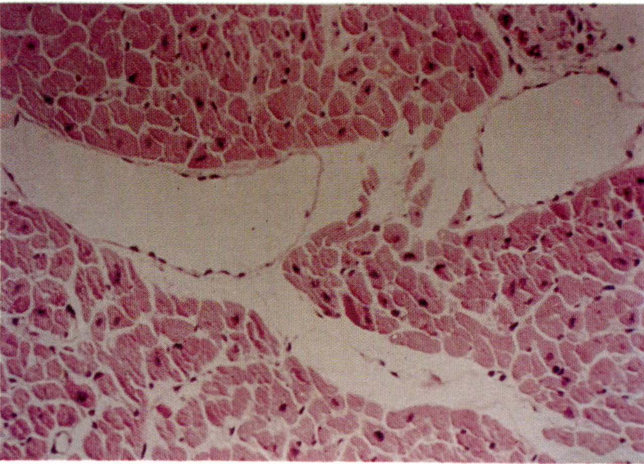

Figure 37

Figure 35. The disappearance of regular cardiac muscle cell nuclei is occurring simultaneously with the lysis of the muscle fibers near the epicardial surface. Within the lysing muscle fibers appear tiny, hyperchromatic, dedifferentiated nuclei (B). These nuclei may have the potential for the development of Type B Aschoff cells as well as new cardiac muscle fibers and possibly new connective tissue fibers (as will be explained by photomicrographs later in this chapter). The sarcolemma of the lysed muscle cell is faintly detectable (arrow). H&E x 400

Figure 36. In a cleft-like space created by lysis of cardiac muscle fibers, tiny hyperchromatic dedifferentiated nuclei as shown in the previous figure are noted. Some of the nuclei have not yet been cleared of remnants of lysing muscle elements. Note that there are several similar tiny nuclei at the periphery of the partially damaged surrounding muscle fibers. H&E x 382

Figure 36-1. In this case of fulminating acute rheumatic fever, extensive myocardial lysis is producing wide cleft or sinus-like spaces filled with mostly clear fluid. In the lumen of a sinus an arrow points to dangling incompletely dissolved myofibers of peripheral cardiac muscle. The endothelium and the content of two vascular channels (A and B) are dissolving from the product of muscle lysis. Rare Aschoff nodules were found only after extensive searching. H&E x 90

Figure 37. This figure shows two wide channels containing clear fluid and lined by a delicate fibrillary membrane. Tiny nuclei in parts of this membrane are arranged linearly in preparation to develop an endothelial membrane. (Channels containing clear fluid at this stage are usually called lymphatic channels.) Note that the incomplete lysis of cardiac muscle between the two developing vascular channels is probably preventing their unification. Also note the appearance of an Aschoff body adjacent to the vascular channel in the upper right corner. Such close association of Aschoff bodies with vascular channels, as in this figure and in figure 37-1, is probably the reason behind one theory that Aschoff bodies arise from peripheral vascular connective tissue. H&E x 260

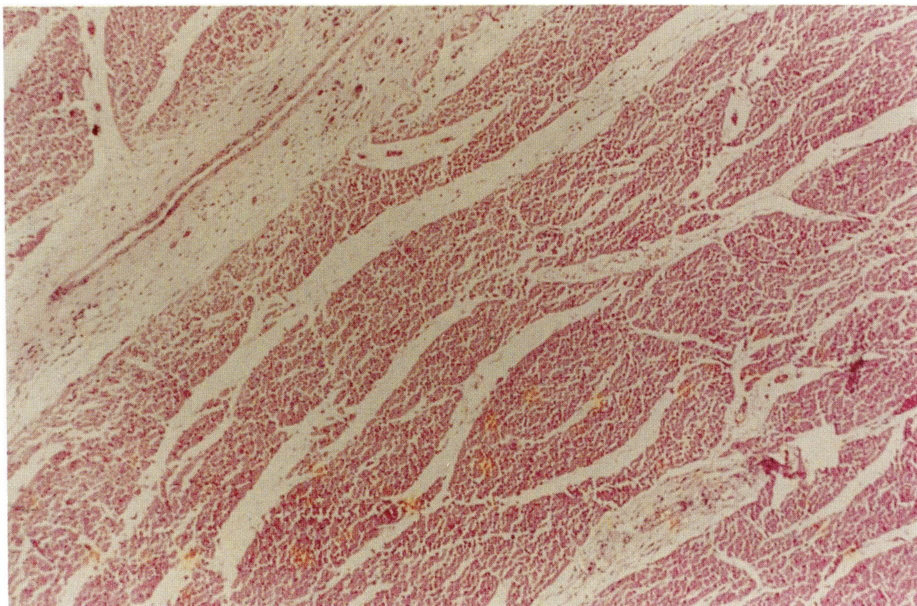

Figure 37-1.

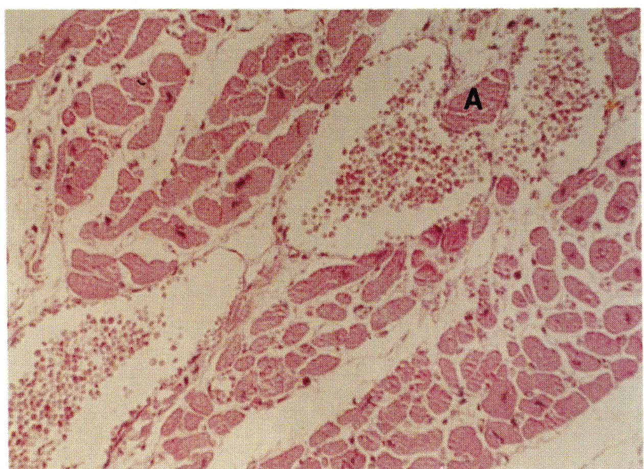

Figure 37-2.

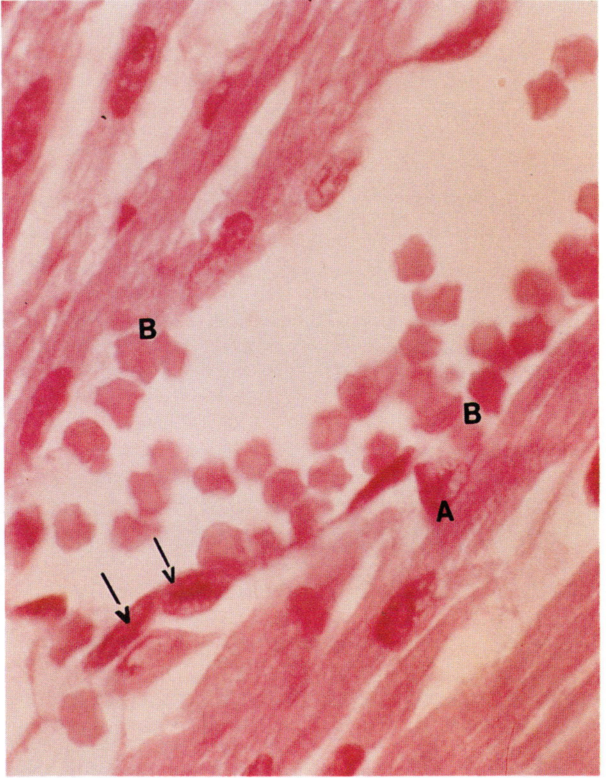

Figure 37-3.

Figure 37-1. This figure demonstrates a large number of Aschoff bodies at the peripheral part of a well developed blood vessel. Both the Aschoff bodies and vascular channels are products of the lysis of cardiac muscle (as shown here). In the first two chapters vascular channel formation from cardiac lysis is explained. H&E x 45

Figure 37-2. This picture depicts two wide blood capillaries occupying the space created by and out of muscle lysis. Upon careful examination, one can see that red cells are developing from the background remnants of granular lysing muscle. These remnants are presented as red particles of various sizes and shades (compare with figs. 11-2 and 13-1). (A) points to a whole muscle fiber resisting lysis. H&E x 140

Figure 37-3. This figure demonstrates the possibility of development of Anitschkow myocytes from cardiac muscle in a non-rheumatic heart. Blood and blood vessel development from cardiac muscle, already described in chapter one, is also presented here. In this figure the participation of Anitschkow myocytes of cardiac muscle origin (arrows) together with the elongated cardiac muscle nucleus are taking part in the development of an endothelial wall. Anitschkow myocytes (A) as well as red cells (B) are developing from dissolving muscle fibers. H&E x 1312

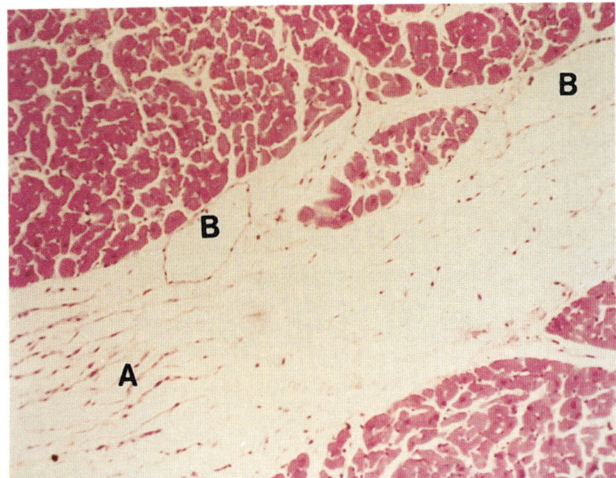

Figure 38

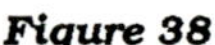

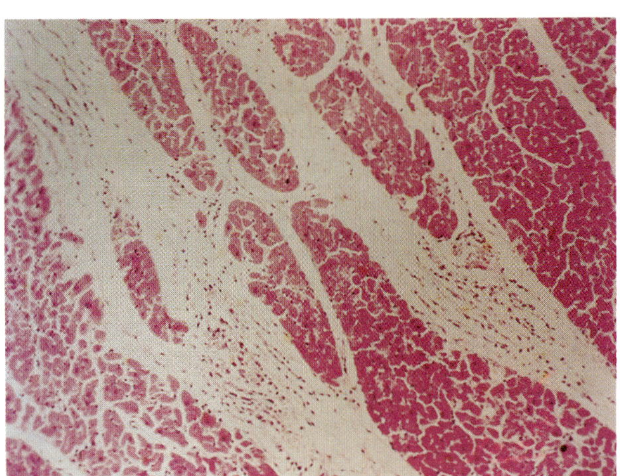

Figure 39

Figure 38. Shown here are the preliminary stages of repair of a wide cleft of lysed muscle by a delicate net-like formation of fine fibrils in association with tiny dedifferentiated cells. (This formation often precedes, in favorable conditions, sarcolemma formation followed by the development of regular cardiac muscle fibers; see figure 42.) In the lower left quadrant a concentration of these cells, along with the developing fibrils in a linear, parallel arrangement, is shown as an early stage of spindle-shaped Aschoff body (A) formation. Note: two capillaries (B) arising from muscle lysis and lined with delicate membranes containing sparse, tiny, dedifferentiated nuclei. H&E x 78

Figure 39. This is a low magnification view of different stages of formation of spindle-shaped Aschoff bodies. This formation occurred in the space derived from muscle lysis and through the stages shown in figures 36 and 38. H&E x 58

Figure 40. Further development of a spindle-shaped Aschoff body from the previous stages as shown in figures 36, 38 and 39 is presented here. The shaggy developing cytoplasm of Type B Aschoff cells gives the appearance of what is known as fibrinoid material (a). The origin of striated cardiac muscle as a further development from this stage (fibrinoid material) is better viewed in figures 42-45. The remaining area of the original pathway of muscle lysis has become narrowed due to faster muscle regeneration from dedifferentiated cells within the already formed network of sarcolemma (similar to that shown in figure 38). An (arrow) points to a new group of fully developed muscle fibers with regular muscle cell nuclei. The above processes are believed to be the normal way of muscle regeneration. Compare the muscle

developed by these regular regenerative processes with the atypical regenerative processes taking place within the Aschoff body. H&E x 95

Figure 41. This is a magnified view of the lower right area of figure 40, including a part of the same group of newly formed muscle fibers, which is shown in the upper left corner of this figure. Dedifferentiated cells (a) can be seen along the margin of the remaining peripheral muscle bundles and in the center of this figure. Further developing muscle cells or myoblasts (b) are shown along the margin and inside the original cleft area. (c) shows a segment of regenerating striated sarcoplasm (the use of a magnifying glass would be helpful). H&E x 503

Figure 42. Regeneration of muscle fibers (A) is occurring inside the Aschoff body which has been developed through Type B cytogenesis following myocardial lysis. (B) points to a myofiber formed in the normal way within the newly formed sarcolemma outside the Aschoff body. H&E x 486

4. Further verification of atypical ways of regeneration of cardiac muscle fibers with cross striations within Aschoff bodies using special stains for the identification of muscle (figs. 43-45)

Figures 43, 44 and 45. Each of these photomicrographs of Aschoff bodies illustrates regeneration of cardiac muscle fibers (A's) with cross striations by application of special stains for identification of muscle element. Figure 43, Phosphotungstic acid-hematoxylin stain x 503; figure 44, Verhoeff van Gieson stain x 370; and figure 45, Masson's trichrome stain x 410

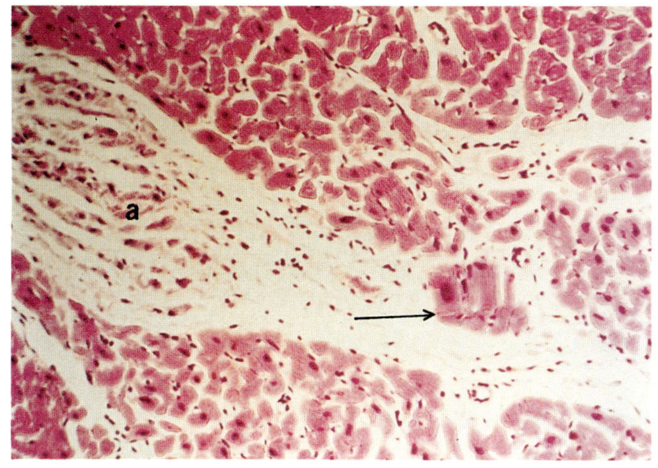

Figure 40

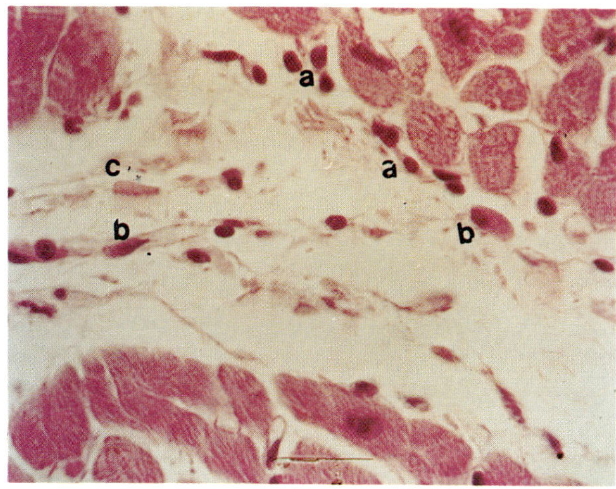

Figure 41

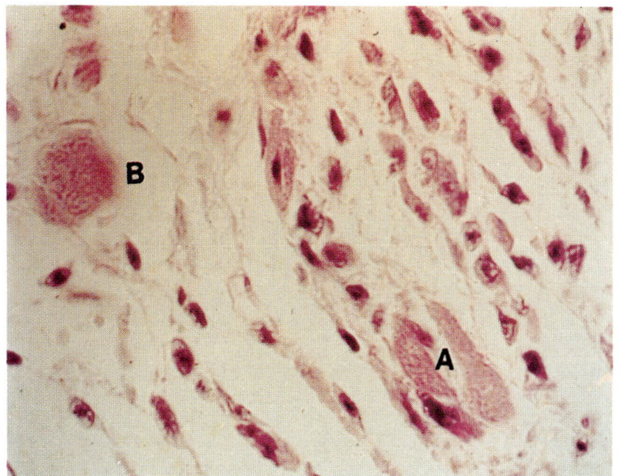

Figure 42

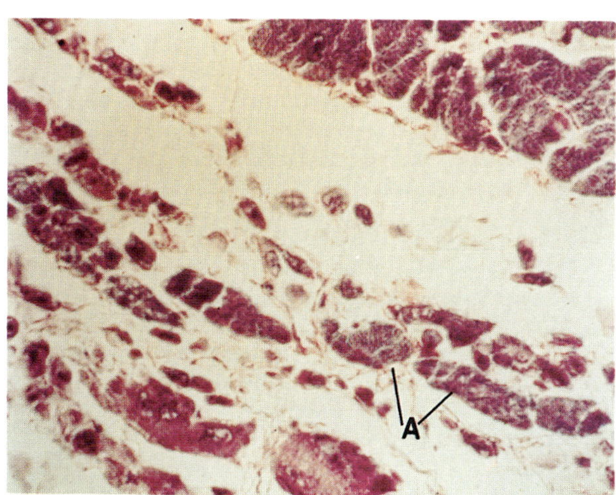

Figure 43

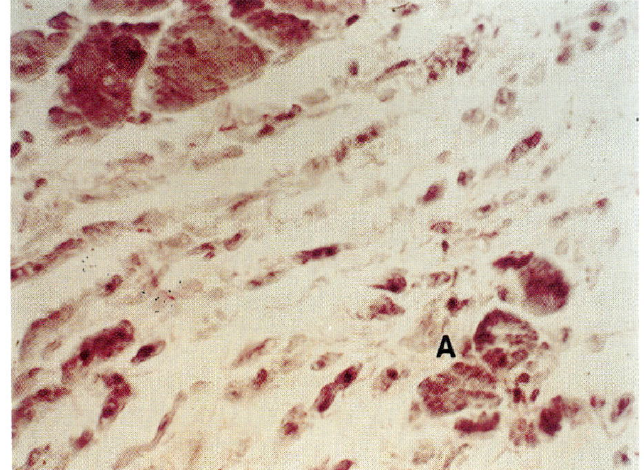

Figure 44

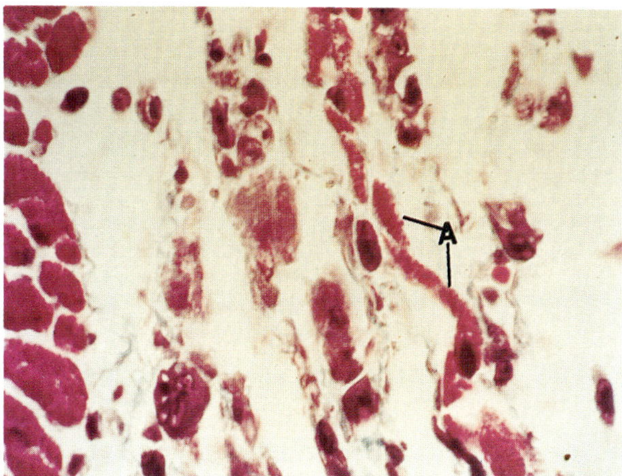

Figure 45

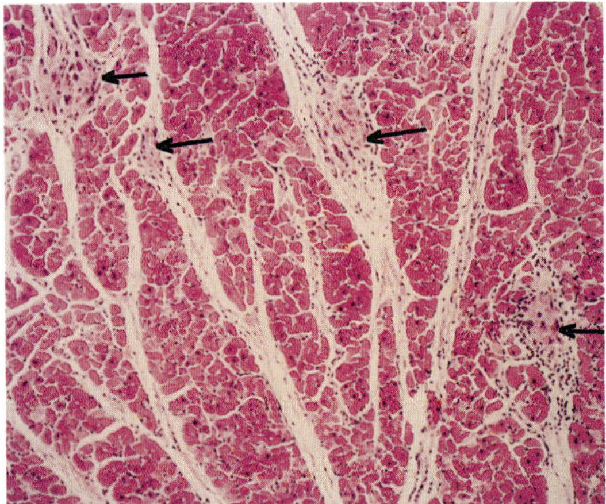

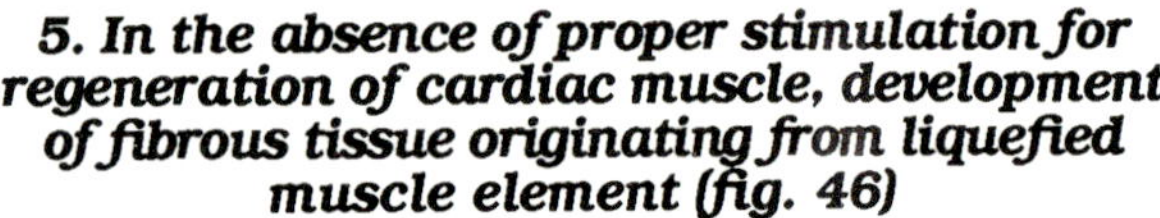

Figure 46

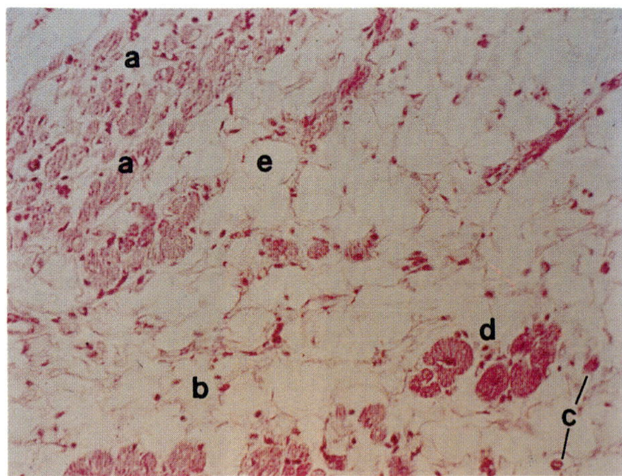

Figure 47

5. In the absence of proper stimulation for regeneration of cardiac muscle, development of fibrous tissue originating from liquefied muscle element (fig. 46)

Figure 46. This figure shows Aschoff bodies (arrows) lying in the path of narrow fibrous septae which are replacing the original tracts of myocardial lysis. (In another area, figures 35 and 36, from the same section acute myocardial lysis is taking place with production of cleft-like spaces.) Note: many tiny dedifferentiated nuclei, some appearing as lymphocytes, are arising from damaged muscle fibers particularly at the periphery of Aschoff bodies on the right. H&E x 70

6. Cellular lysis involving individual muscle fibers with retention of sarcolemma (myocytolysis) and possible regeneration of muscle fibers within retained sarcolemma (fig. 47) and possible origin of Aschoff body (fig. 48) as shown in outer myocardium

Figure 47. This is subepicardial cardiac muscle showing various phases of cellular lysis mostly with the retention of sarcolemma. (a) shows degenerating muscle fibers undergoing lysis; and (b) an area where faintly stained sarcolemma and a few newly developed dedifferentiated cardiac cells are seen. Compare (b) with figures 26 (B) and 35 (B). (c) shows developing muscle cells within retained sarcolemma. Bundles of newly and fully formed cardiac muscle fibers are shown at (d). Compare the better staining quality and the shape of these newly formed muscle fibers having cross striations with the degenerating muscle fibers in (a) and other areas. (e) illustrates an area where the sarcolemma assumes a rounded appearance. In the absence of stimulus for muscle regeneration it is possible that intracellular fat infiltration may occur. Upon casual observation, one may easily mistake the microscopic findings shown here as infiltra-

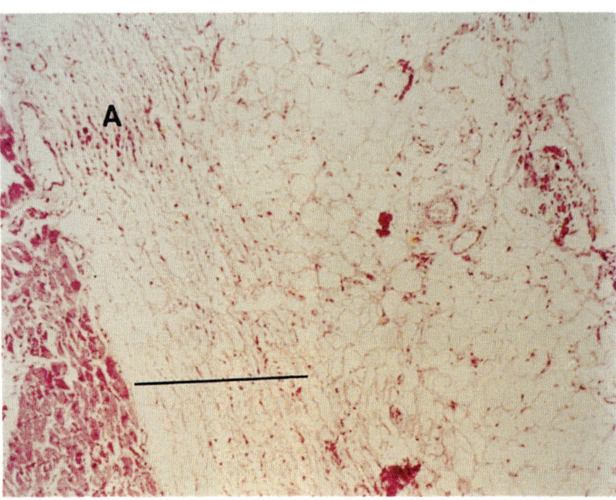

Figure 48

tion of normal cardiac muscle fibers instead of fat replacement of damaged muscle fibers. H&E x 61

Figure 48. Extensive damage of subepicardial myocardium is shown in the outer two-thirds of this figure. Such changes give a gross appearance of watery, translucent gelatinous pericardium. The right half of this photomicrograph shows intracellular lysis of sarcoplasm (myocytolysis) which simulates adipose tissue. The middle one-fourth (line) shows cellular lysis with partial retention of collapsed sarcolemma. The above area shows many tiny dedifferentiated cells. The early stages of spindle-shaped Aschoff body formation are seen at (A). Such findings as shown here may give a wrong conclusion that Aschoff nodules are arising from subepicardial fatty tissue to casual observers. (See figures 36, 38 and 39 for further development of such Aschoff bodies.) H&E x 54

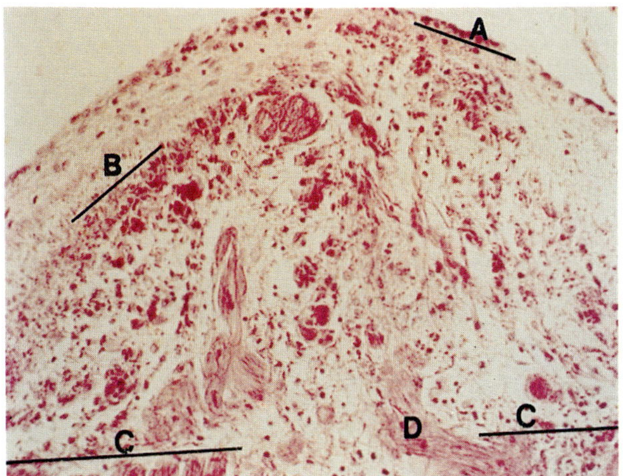

Figure 49

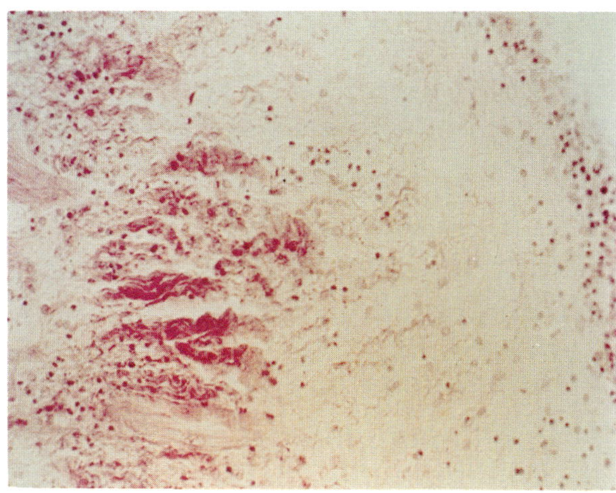

Figure 50

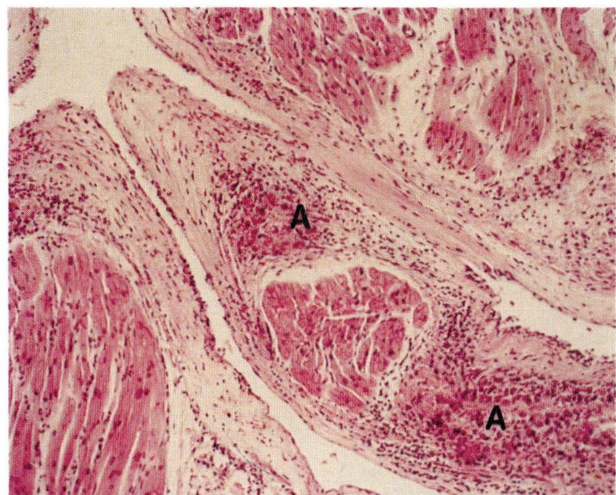

Figure 51

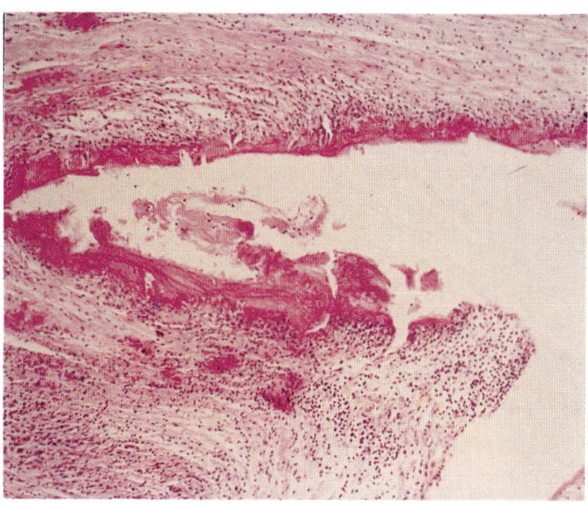

Figure 52

7. Extensive fibrillary and fibrinoid degeneration of muscle fibers in the process of development of thickened fibrous endocardium (figs. 49-50)

Figure 49. This figure demonstrates extensive fibrinoid and fibrillary degeneration of subendocardial cardiac muscle in conjunction with the development of thickened endocardium. Inward progression of this process is demarcated by lines A, B and C. A few intact muscle fibers can be identified in these degenerating areas. Line A is just beneath the endocardial lining cells. Thickened endocardium has already formed to the left of line B. Line (C) points to further progression of demarcation zone between myocardium and developing thickened subendocardium. The demarcation plane is free from muscle fibers except for a small area (D). No Aschoff body formation can be seen in this figure. H&E x 150

Figure 50. Wavy fibrillary material derived from degenerated muscle can be seen close to the inner border of the cardiac wall. Compare this fibrillary change with that of individual muscle fibers seen in figure 30 (g). H&E x 140

8. Acute inflammatory reaction of papillary muscle (fig. 51), and the mitral valve (figs. 52 and 53); Anitschkow myocytes arising from myogenic fibrous tissue of mitral valve (fig. 54) act as mother cells of many of the inflammatory cells (fig. 53)

(Figs. 53 and 54 are magnified views of two different points in fig. 52)

Figure 51. Intense inflammatory reaction associated with cardiac muscle degeneration and Aschoff body formation (A) is shown in the papillary muscle of the cardiac valves. (Various inflammatory cells that may arise from cardiac muscle, other than Anitschkow myocytes and their derivatives, are shown in detail in chapter four.) This acute inflammatory reaction results in fibrous thickening of the endocardium. H&E x 85

Figure 52. This view of the mitral valve shows an acute inflammatory reaction and deposition of fibrin. (See the magnified view of inflammatory cells in figure 53 and origin of Anitschkow myocytes in collagenous fibrous tissue of the heart valve fig. 54.) H&E x 55

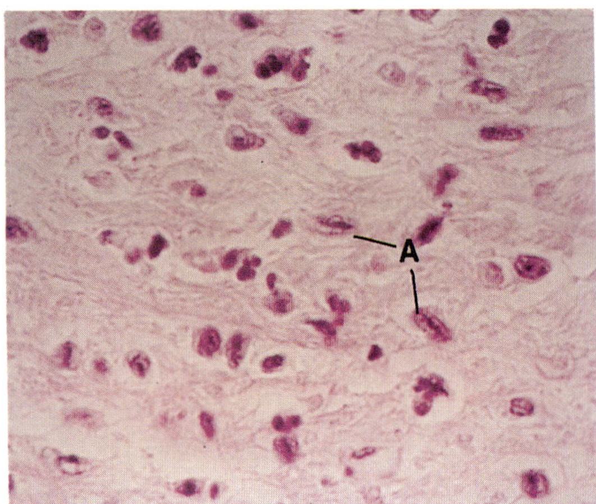

Figure 53

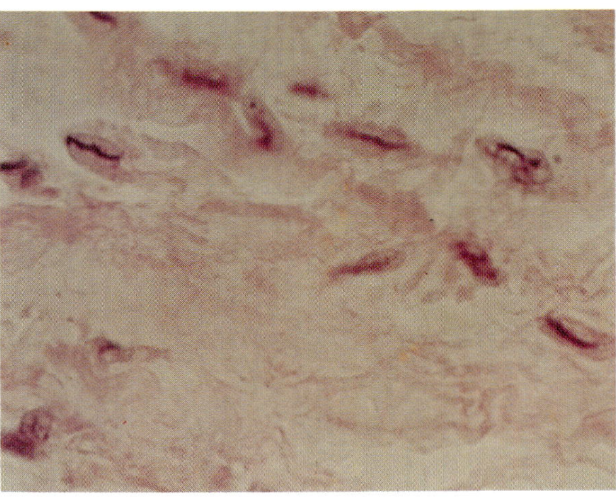

Figure 54

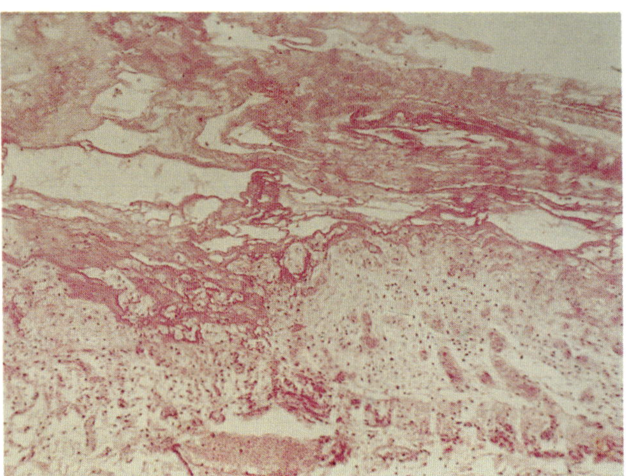

Figure 55

Figure 53. Presented here is a magnified view of the inflammatory reaction of the cardiac valve shown in figure 52 in low magnification. Note the inflammatory cells are composed of several well-defined Anitschkow myocytes (A), and many highly irregular nuclear structures with somewhat similar nuclear patterns showing their origin from Anitschkow myocytes. H&E x 600

Figure 54. This figure depicts the origin of Anitschkow myocytes from the fibrillary collagenous tissue of cardiac valves shown in figure 52. Since the cardiac valves are derived embryologically from cardiac muscle (see figures 22-1 and 22-2) the fibrous tissue of valves shows the same capacity as cardiac muscle in production of Anitschkow myocytes. H&E x 560

9. Prominent serofibrinous pericarditis, an occasional complication of acute rheumatic fever (fig. 55)

Figure 55. To roughly complete the presentation of various cardiac complications associated with acute rheumatic fever, this photomicrograph of serofibrinous pericarditis has been included without further explanation. H&E x 55

CHAPTER FOUR
DAMAGE AND TRANSFORMATION OF CARDIAC MUSCLE IN CORONARY OCCLUSION FROM A SINGLE CASE STUDY

In coronary occlusion with myocardial infarction, coagulation necrosis of muscle fibers may be followed by the in-situ origin of various reactive cells—histiocytes, 'phagocytes', plasma cells, lymphocytes, segmented nuclear cells, spindle cells, and many unclassified cells—as well as blood and blood capillaries towards the development of granulation tissue and fibrosis. Acute inflammatory exudate and 'hemorrhage' (linked with occasional cardiac rupture) show their origin from ischemic muscle. The development of small and large blood vessels from ischemic muscle is presented as a basis for collateral circulation.

I. INTRODUCTION

The observations presented in this chapter are a detailed study of the cellular changes in the myocardium of a 57-year-old man who died with a diagnosis of recent and acute myocardial infarction caused by coronary occlusion. As seen in this case and discussed here, there are two main types of acute lesions: coagulation necrosis and acute regional suppurative myocarditis. Both of these occurrences are known to be predisposing factors for occasional cardiac rupture (Gould 1960, p. 611).

The first and most commonly known lesion is coagulation necrosis, where muscle fibers become bright-red in color and devoid of striations and nuclei. The different processes of healing from this stage of coagulation necrosis toward formation of collagenous fibrous and vascular tissues are described. The result of the author's detailed study shows that from the infarcted myoplasm, there may directly arise segmented nuclear cells (SN cells), plasma cells, lymphocytes, monocytes, histiocytes, 'phagocytes', spindle cells with collagenous fibrils, blood, and blood vessels. Such developmetal processes are presented here with photomicrographs from the myocardium of the same patient. What is usually known as hemorrhage is found to be the profuse development of red cells from freshly infarcted muscle which has undergone coagulation necrosis.

The second, a less emphasized effect of coronary occlusion, is found to be acute myocarditis of unknown etiology. This acute inflammatory reaction almost similar to acute suppurative inflammation occurs with a preponderance of SN cells. These cells arise from noninfarcted muscle fibers.

Other cellular changes seen in cardiac muscle in coronary occlusion are: 1. Vacuolar necrosis and vacuolar degeneration of cardiac muscle, usually in close proximity to coagulation necrosis; 2. Suboptimal infarction of muscle fibers with red fibrillary changes The possibility of direct development of fibrosis and large blood vessels from such ischemic muscle tissue is presented; 3. Abnormal nuclear proliferation with development of multinucleated muscle giant cells like tumor giant cells, as nearby altered myoplasm produces plasma cells with erythrogenic capability; 4. Altered myoplasm may also show proliferation of nuclei like those of foreign body giant cells.

II. BRIEF CLINICAL HISTORY AND FINAL POSTMORTEM DIAGNOSIS OF THE CASE USED IN THIS STUDY
(as copied from the original autopsy protocol)

A 57-year-old man was admitted to the hospital complaining of shortness of breath and occasional chest pain. One month earlier he was hospitalized with evidence of congestive heart failure associated with engorged neck veins and hepatosplenomegaly. It was believed that the patient was having an extension of a previous infarction and also a new infarction, as suggested clinically by the signs and symptoms, cardiac enzymes, and electrocardiogram studies. White blood cell count was 13,550 with 78% segmented neutrophils. The patient expired five days later. (The autopsy was completed within three hours of death. The prosector was the author during her residency period at the St. Louis City Hospital in 1953.)

The final diagnosis:

1. Arteriosclerotic heart disease with severe coronary arteriosclerosis:
   a) Thrombotic occlusion of the anterior descending and circumflex branch of the left coronary artery;
   b) Recent anterolateral infarcts including interventricular septum;
   c) Cardiomegaly 500 gms.;
   d) Fibrinous pericarditis;
   e) Mural thrombi of the left ventricle.

2. Marked passive congestion of the liver and spleen.
3. Congestion and edema of the lungs.
4. Recent infarcts of the right kidney.

Thirty years later, the detailed reexamination of a duplicate set of slides of myocardium, which were saved for future study, reveal the following histopathogenesis processes.

III. MICROSCOPIC FINDINGS OF COAGULATION NECROSIS OF CARDIAC MUSCLES IN CORONARY OCCLUSION

The successive stages towards healing with fibrosis from coagulation necrosis of cardiac muscle are described in figures 56-70. The necrotic muscle fibers may show granular fragmentation with the appearance of basophilic particles (figure 59). For possible further development from this stage to the development of red cells, as well as the beginning stages of development of some other inflammatory cells, see figure 72. From dissolving muscle fibers (which have undergone coagulation necrosis) one may see the origin of cells commonly called 'phagocytes'. These cells are demonstrated in longitudinal planes (figs. 60 and 61), and in transverse planes of the muscle fibers (figs. 62 and 73). The nuclei of these cells may first appear as tiny chromatin dots (fig. 60) and the cytoplasm is carved out from the dissolved myoplasm. When red cells are formed from the cytoplasm of these cells, the latter are commonly designated as 'erythrophagocytes' (fig. 73) instead of erythrogenic cells.

Figures 63-65 demonstrate early reparative stages of infarcted muscle with development of spindle-shaped nuclei, possibly in precollagenous background. Infarcted myofibers 'in mass' may transform into a bluishgrey, somewhat opaque ground glass-like substance (fig. 65) before giving rise to spindle cells, various mononuclear cells, and blood capillaries.

One may see the direct development from infarcted muscle (in early coagulation necrosis state) of various cells falling under the category of spindle cells, and many mononuclear reactive cells (particularly plasma cells) in addition to blood and blood vessels (figs. 66 and 83). Further progression from this stage (fig. 67) towards healing with fibrosis and vascularization is shown successively in figures 68 to 70. These figures show successive transformation of plasma cells into spindle cells with collagenous fibrous background, as well as blood capillary formation.

Brown pigment derived from the infarcted myoplasm and associated with different nuclear structures, usually designated as 'macrophages/phagocytes' is shown in figures 61 and 69. A larger area of coagulation necrosis leading towards granulation tissue formation is shown in figure 71. Findings corresponding to these were found by Yanagisawa-Miwa et al (1992) during a study of infarcted myocardium.

Blood present in the infarcted muscle (figs. 74 and 75) commonly described as 'hemorrhage' is found to be myogenic in origin. This profuse red cell development from infarcted heart muscle is compared with a similar development from ischemic or infarcted liver parenchyma (fig. 76) of this patient having congestive heart failure. (Fig. 13-1 reveals how quickly and how extensively liver parenchyma may be converted into large developing blood vessels under extreme anoxic conditions as shown in an asphyxiated rabbit.)

IV. ACUTE REGIONAL MYOCARDITIS WITH FIBRINOUS PERICARDITIS
(another important finding of coronary occlusion)

In areas of acute myocarditis with unknown etiology (figs. 77-81), the reactive cells are found to arise from cardiac muscle fibers (figs. 77 and 78). The predominant cells are segmented nuclear cells. Other cells include eosinophils, plasma cells, lymphocytes, and spindle cells. In the inflamed area, blood and blood vessels may form directly from cardiac muscles (figs. 78 and 79). Also the segmented nuclear cells of muscle origin take an active part in red cell formation. These reactive cells by their enzymatic activity may enhance the liquefaction process of muscle with possible cardiac rupture, a fatal complication of myocardial infarction (Gould 1960, p. 612). Rupture of cardiac muscle may also occur by hemmorhage, which is found to be profuse blood formation with replacement of muscle tissue. Edmonson and Hoxie (1942) found that among 865 hearts with untreated infarcts due to coronary artery disease there were 72 instances of spontaneous rupture.

In some ways, dissolution of acutely inflamed outer cardiac muscle may produce a magenta-colored (in H&E stain) hemoglobin gel-like substance and participate in the deposition of fibrin on the surface (figs. 77, 80 and 81), thus causing what is known as fibrinous pericarditis.

V. OTHER LESS EMPHASIZED MICROSCOPIC CHANGES ASSOCIATED WITH ACUTE AND RECENT MYOCARDIAL INFARCTION CAUSED BY CORONARY OCCLUSION

In addition to coagulation necrosis and acute myocarditis with fibrinous pericarditis as stated above, other less emphasized microscopic changes seen in the heart with coronary occlusion are as follows:

1. Vacuolar necrosis and vacuolar degeneration

Vaculolar necrosis (fig. 82) may be described as aseptic and noncoagulation necrosis associated with swiss cheese like vacuole formation. Both the sarcoplasmic characteristics and the muscle cell nuclei disappear in early stages. This gives a bland and friable look with no evidence of muscle tissue. The possibility of blood formation from such muscle tissues is shown in figure 82.

Vacuolar degeneration (figs. 83 and 84) may also be present in myocardium showing nearby coagulation necrosis. Vacuolar degeneration has been emphasized by Schlesinger and Reiner (1955). This type of degeneration is different from the lysis of individual muscle fibers with retention of sarcolemma (myocytolysis) as shown in the myocardium in acute rheumatic fever (fig.47). Also shown is the possibility of regeneration of myofibers from dedifferentiated lymphocyte-like cells which are arising in lysing myofibers; this is demonstrated in McDonald (1957 and 1975a) and in the third chapter of this volume.

From vacuolar degenerated muscle one may see the development of blood, blood capillaries, and chronic reactive cells—mainly plasma cells and lymphocytes. In vacuolar degeneration, cardiac muscle fibers retain their nuclear and myoplasmic characteristics (figs. 83 and 84) for a longer period.

2. Ischemic myofibers in sub-optimal coagulation necrosis stage acting as a possible source of direct development of fibrosis and development of large blood vessels

Such myofibers with loss of striations and consisting of red fibrillary structures soon lose the red stain and become fine spindle cells in a somewhat collagenous background (fig. 85). The possibility of development of large blood vessels from such ischemic myocardial tissue as shown in figures 86 and 87 may be considered in development of collateral circulation.

3. Ischemic myofibers producing muscle giant cells like tumor giant cells and also generating plasma cells with capacity to form blood and blood capillaries

It is not rare to find individual muscle fibers producing large nuclei often clumped together, known as muscle giant cells (figs. 88) like tumor giant cells. From these ischemic myofibers, the origin of tiny plasma cell bodies and their maturation toward plasma cells with formation of blood and blood capillaries can be seen.

4. Origin of multiple nuclei like those of foreign body giant cells from hyalinized basophilic myoplasm

Multiple nuclei may start as almost invisible structures in a faintly stained homogeneous lightly basophilic background of altered myoplasm from which regular cardiac muscle nuclei and cross striation have already disappeared (figs. 89 and 90).

VI. SUMMARY AND SHORT COMMENT

It has been demonstrated through the photomicrographs that all types of inflammatory/reactive cells (including those cells which are known as phagocytes) as well as blood, blood vessels and fibrous tissue may be derived locally from myofibers. These myofibers, the mother cells, may be apparently normal or damaged muscles, including those which have undergone infarction. The development of red cells occurs directly as hemoglobin globules from myofibers (intact or damaged) and even from the product of muscle necrosis. Similarly, segmented nuclear cells, lymphocytes, plasma cells, and less defined cells (such as histiocytes, monocytes, and phagocytes) are also shown to arise locally from cardiac muscle or muscle product and to have erythrogenic capacity. In Vol. I, the author describes the possibility of development of red cells directly as hemoglobin globules from various benign and malignant cells, and also from every type of inflammatory cell in benign and malignant tissues. The presence of erythrocytes within inflammatory cells has been sporadically mentioned by others [Smith (1958), Marin-Padilla (1977), Rigsdall, et al, (1979), Hernandez and Steane (1984)] and others, but generally such an occurrence has been categorized as 'erythrophagocytosis.'

It is a common practice to refer to blood seen outside the blood vessel (figs. 74 and 75) as 'hemorrhage', even though there is no evidence of ruptured vessels or scattered red cells over the tissues. The root of this deduction probably lies in the fact that the local development of blood is generally unthinkable at the present time.

Acute regional myocarditis of unknown etiology and associated with myocardial infarction (as described in this chapter) is like a suppurative inflammation affecting cardiac muscle. On careful examination one will see that apparently regular muscle fibers are being replaced, mostly by developing segmented nuclear cells. Various developmental stages of acute inflammatory cells are demonstrated in figures 78 and 79. These changes start within muscle fibers as minute groups of chromatin particles and then progress towards formation of segmented nuclei, while the cytoplasm is derived from the lysing myoplasm. The erythrogenic capacity of these newly formed SN cells is demonstrated in figure 79. There are many examples in Vol. I of narrow columns of locally developed segmented nuclear cells arising from benign and malignant tissues, and their transformation into columns of red cells in development of narrow blood capillaries. A similar observation is made by the author on local development of plasma cells and their erythrogenic capacity either directly or indirectly through intermediary reactive cells of plasma cell origin as described earlier (McDonald, 1989). In this chapter it is shown that plasma cells of cardiac muscle origin are directly producing blood and capillary walls (figs. 67 and 88). The common supposition that inflammatory cells are derived only in bone marrow and are carried to the inflamed area by circulating blood probably has obscured the fact that inflammatory cells are derived locally as shown here.

In addition, from ischemic myocardium the production of new and sometimes large blood vessels (figs. 86 and 87) may explain the possible mechanism in development of collateral circulation in cases of coronary stenosis or occlusion.

The author admits that she has not studied the possibility of regeneration of cardiac muscle in myocardial infarction. The reader will find ample evidence for regeneration of cardiac muscle in the chapter on acute rheumatic fever.

VII. EXPLANATION OF FIGURES

The photomicrographs (figs. 56-90) are taken from the autopsy specimen of a patient whose clinical history is described earlier in this chapter (see page 63). All figures are from the ventricular wall with the exception of figure 76, which is from the liver of the same patient. Hematoxylin and eosin stain is used in each figure.

1. Acute myocardial infarction causing coagulation necrosis (fig.56); and the subsequent development (figs. 57-75)

Figure 56. The central portion of this figure shows a fresh myocardial infarction characterized by the presence of bright red discolored muscle tissue. Note that the surrounding thick band of subendocardial myocardium is not affected by coronary occlusion. It is usually believed that the inner myocardium has additional nutrition from the blood in the cardiac lumen (Gould 1960, p. 602). For details see figure 58 where the area 56 (A) is shown in higher magnification. H&E x 52

Figure 57. Here in the outer myocardium coagulation necrosis assumes a different character as opposed to what is shown in figures 56 and 58. The gradual changes of infarcted muscle towards production of what is commonly known as serous atrophy of the pericardium is shown in three segments A, B and C, from right to left. The blotchy purplish appearance of necrosed muscle with absence of striations and nuclei, and the presence of a few fine basophilic pyknotic particles, occupy a triangular zone in the upper right section (A). Adjacent to the left border of this triangle is an obliquely lying narrow segment (B) of infarcted muscle, mostly grey with a bleached-out appearance. This area containing minute and sparse nuclear structures is in the process of development towards the next phase (C); here lie thin linear fibrillary elements associated with tiny hyperchromatic nuclei and forming a mesh-like structure enclosing clear spaces. In gross examination of the heart such an area would give a translucent gelatinous appearance which is commonly known as serous atrophy of the pericardium. It is conceivable that under favorable conditions fat may accumulate in such mesh-like structures in development of subepicardial fat. H&E x 130

Figure 58. This is a higher magnification of area (A) in figure 56. The infarcted area is beginning to extend into the adjoining muscle fibers as demonstrated by the appearance of speckled bright red color (a) in the muscle fibers. With the disappearance of a certain amount of fully infarcted myoplasm through dissolution, more gaps appear between the remaining infarcted myofibers. H&E x 520

Figure 59. Fragmentation and reddish grey discoloration of the infarcted hypertrophic myofibers are prominently seen. Note in this area the appearance of tiny, blue-stained, scattered particles. H&E x 520

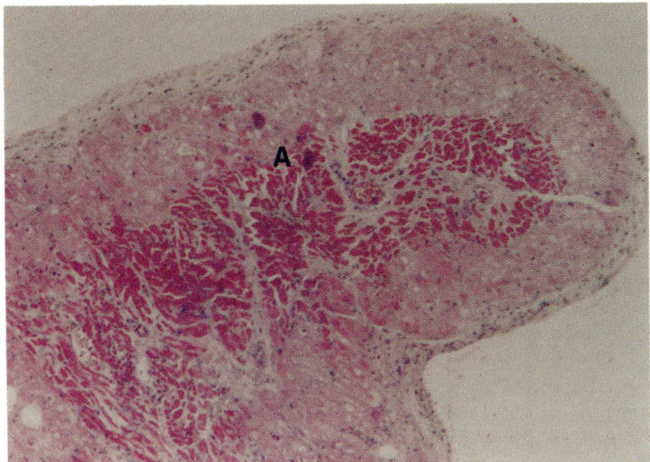

Figure 56

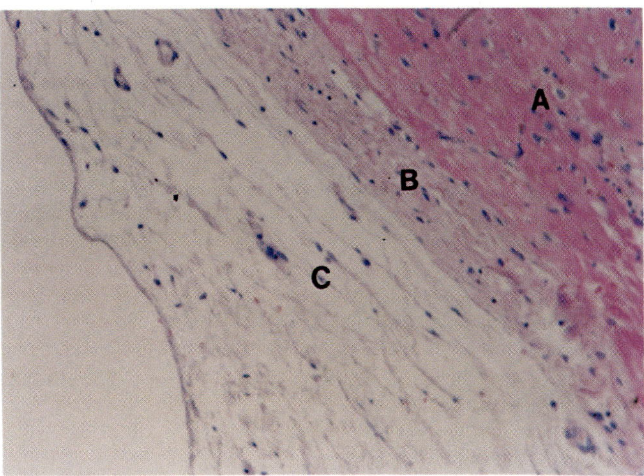

Figure 57

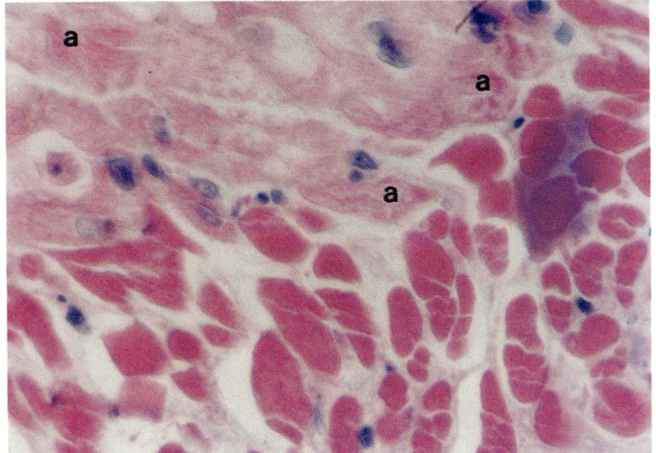

Figure 58

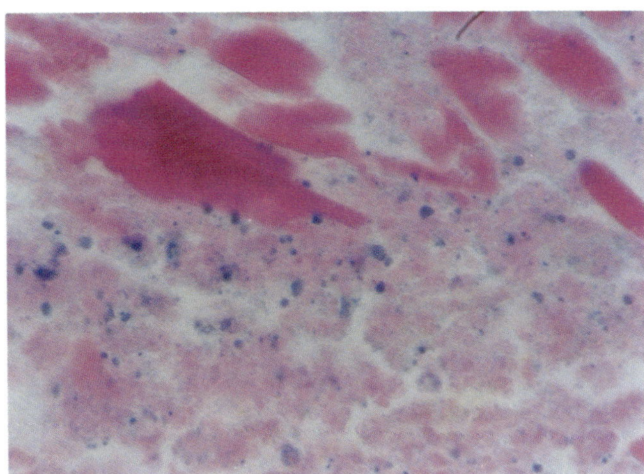

Figure 59

From infarcted myofibers the origin of histiocytes/phagocytes presented in longitudinal planes (figs. 60 and 61), and in transverse planes (figs. 62, 63 and 73)

From infarcted myofibers, the origin of other reactive cells such as lymphocytes, plasma cells, monocytes, and spindle cells toward fibrosis (figs. 61-70)

Figure 60. Partially dissolving infarcted muscle fibers changing from bright red to pinkish-grey are shown here in longitudinal planes. Within the dissolving muscle fibers, large cells with tiny nuclei of variable sizes are arising. These are usually categorized as 'phagocytes.' The cytoplasm of these cells (a) is formed by carving out the infarcted muscle element. Note the shade of brownish color developing in the cytoplasm of these histiocytes. Note also the appearance of tiny hyperchromatic nuclear structures (b) in the dissolving muscle fibers. H&E x 260

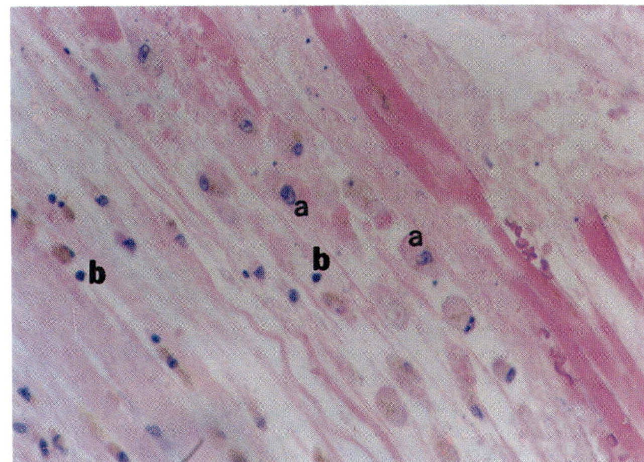

Figure 60

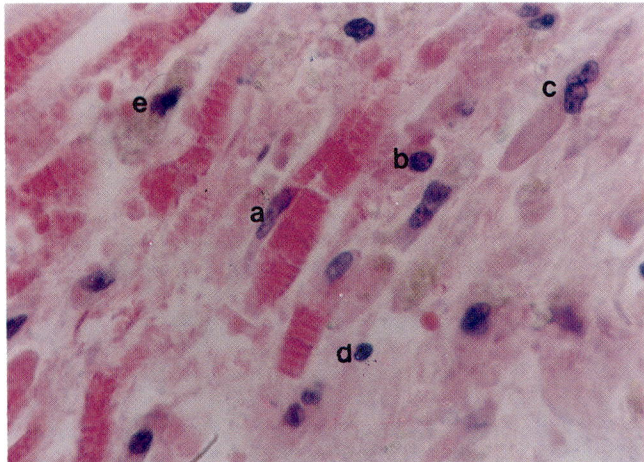

Figure 61

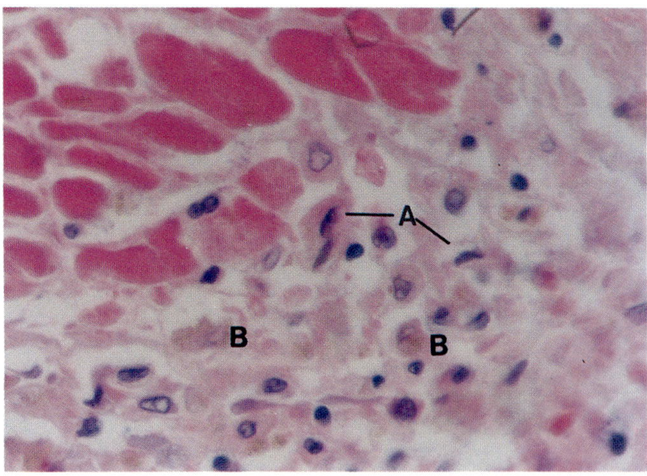

Figure 62

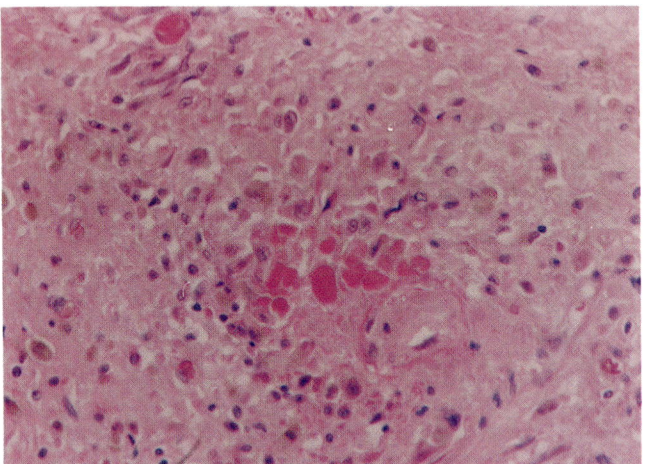

Figure 63

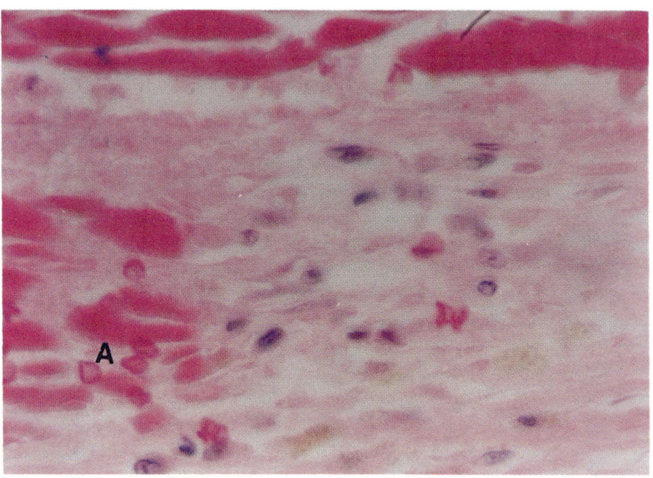

Figure 64

Figure 61. The red infarcted myofibers (some of which contain swollen transverse parallel striations) are changing into a pinkish-brownish-grey color and are partially dissolved. Within this altered remaining myoplasm there appear nuclei of different shapes such as: (a) an elongated narrow nucleus, (b) a round nucleus in an eccentric position simulating a plasma cell, (c) a large, irregular multilobed nucleus, (d) a tiny lymphocyte-like nucleus, and (e) a large irregular nucleus with brown pigment granules (usually termed as phagocytes with hemosiderin granules). Somewhat similar changes are shown in figure 62 in a transverse plane of the altered muscle fibers. H&E x 520

Figure 62. Arising from the changing infarcted muscle fibers are nuclear structures surrounded by the developing cytoplasm derived from infarcted muscle (which is pinkish-brown or pinkish-grey in color). The nuclear structures vary considerably from the tiny hyperchromatic nuclear dots, to that of lymphocyte-like cells, to irregular spindle-shaped nuclei (A). Often these cells, especially the larger cells with irregular nuclei and brownish pigment (B), are customarily termed 'histiocytes/phagocytes'. Compare this figure

with figures 60 and 61 where muscle fibers are shown in the longitudinal planes. H&E x 520

Figure 63. Small portions of the bright red infarcted muscle fibers remain in the center and also near the upper left border of this figure. The remaining area shows further organizational processes compared with the previous figure. Note the irregular spindle-shaped nuclei with ill-defined fibrillary structures (toward development of fibrosis) visible in the upper left and lower right corners. H&E x 260

Prior to nuclear regeneration, frequently seen changes in color and consistency of bright-red infarcted myofibers into pinkish-grey substance (fig. 64); or into bluish-grey, ground glass-like substance (fig. 65)

Figure 64. Here the pinkish-grey substance of infarcted muscle derivatives is giving rise to narrow spindle-shaped nuclei. A few irregularly hemoglobinized red cells can also be seen arising from the infarcted muscle (A). Note the appearance of faintly stained brown pigment in the vanishing infarcted myofibers at right lower segment. H&E x 520

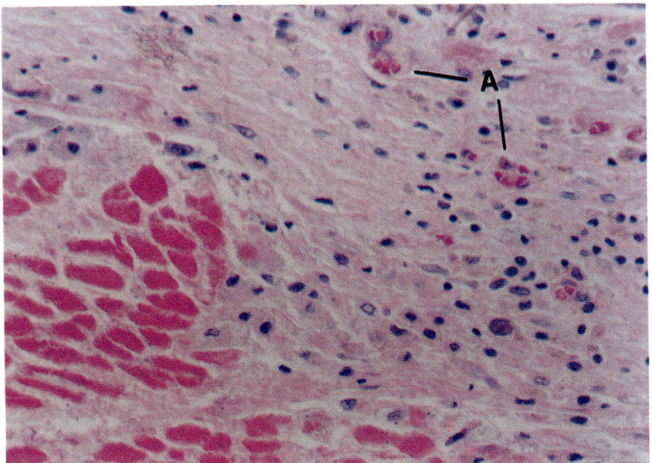

Figure 65

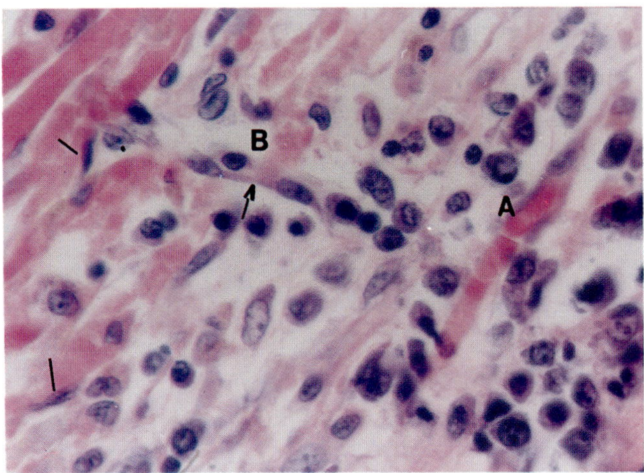

Figure 66

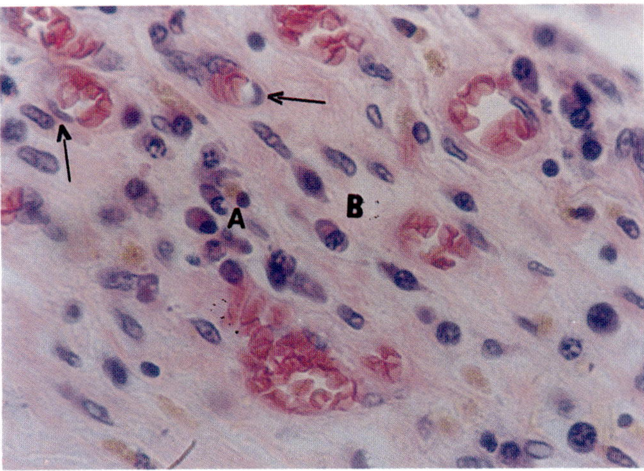

Figure 67

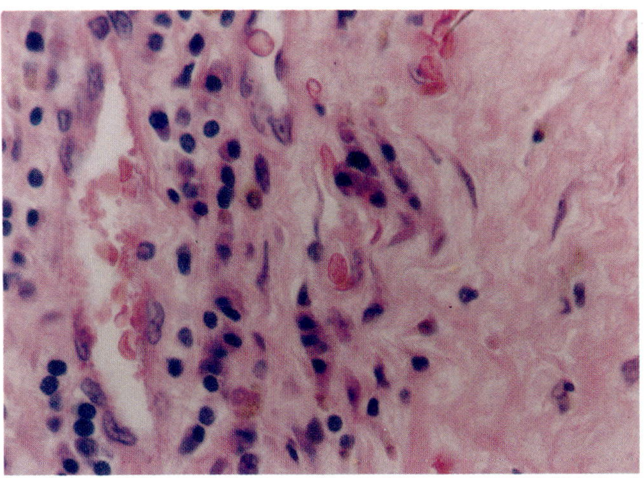

Figure 68

Figure 65. There are many developing small, round, hyperchromatic, lymphocyte-like nuclear structures, some spindle-shaped nuclei, and also several developing blood capillaries (A) all arising from this bluish-grey slate-like background substance derived from infarcted muscle. H&E x 260

From bright red infarcted muscle the possibility of the origin of round mononuclear cells—predominantly plasma cells—and blood capillaries (fig. 66); further developmental stages of plasma cells associated with background substance toward formation of collagenous fibrous tissue (figs. 67-70) and blood capillaries (figs. 67 and 68)

Figure 66. Developmental stages of mononuclear cells, mainly plasma cells of various sizes (see particularly right, lower corner), from infarcted myofibers. A few spindle-shaped nuclei pointed by straight lines, are also developing from the infarcted muscle. On the right, arising from infarcted myoplasm, there is a developing blood capillary (A) with a single column of red cells. On the middle left, across the muscle fibers, there is a suggestion of a developing capillary with endothelium (arrow). (B) points to the

remains of undissolved infarcted myoplasm. H&E x 520

Figure 67. Many plasma cells have started to become spindle cells in the faintly visible fibrillary background, possibly as part of a developing fibrous tissue. A group of tiny plasma cells (A) with tendency for red cell production (erythrogenic plasma cells) lie in continuation with the developing red cell column below. Some plasma cells are becoming spindle cells around (B). From 7, 9, 11 and 1 o'clock positions, developing endothelial cells of local origin (from plasma cells or background substance) can be seen bordering the blood capillaries (arrow). Small clumps of faintly yellowish-brown pigment, some in association with nuclear structures, are scattered throughout the figure. H&E x 520

Progressive stages of healing (from fig. 67) by collagenous fibrous tissue (figs. 68-70) primarily through plasma cells and background substance

Figures 68, 69 and 70. Progressive stages of healing by collagenous fibrous tissue are shown by the transformation of plasma cells into spindle-shaped nuclei through plasmacy-

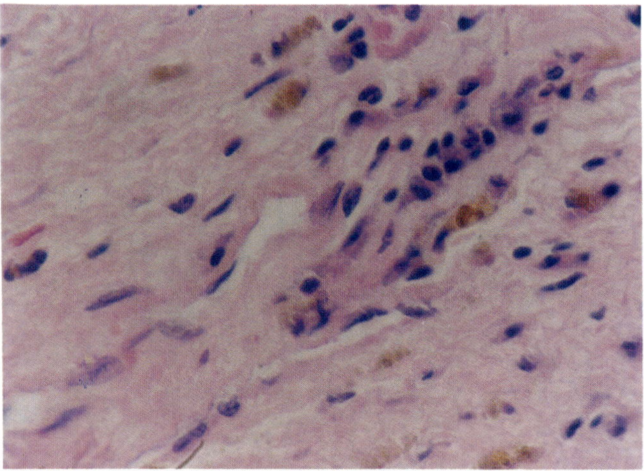

Figure 69

Figure 70

toid cell stages and development of collagenous fibrillary elements from the background substance. The changing cardiac muscle cells with development of intracellular brown pigment granules are commonly designated as phagocytes; such cells are most prominent in figure 69. Figures 68 and 69, H&E x 520; and figure 70, H&E x 130

Covering a wide area, attempted healing processes by infarcted muscle fibers toward fibrosis (fig. 71)
(shown in low magnification)

Figure 71. Bright red infarcted muscle fibers (lying in longitudinal plane) are transforming into what may be called granulation tissue toward fibrosis. H&E x 52

2. The possibility of massive blood formation by infarcted cardiac muscle (figs. 72-75) compared with that of the liver of the same patient (fig. 76)

Development of red cells from the product of infarcted muscle (fig. 72)

Figure 72. On the left, remaining bright red infarcted muscle fibers can still be seen. Arising from fragmented and partially dissolved infarcted muscle, there are red cells of different sizes and of different intensity of red color. H&E x 520

Development of red cells from infarcted myofibers directly and also through erythrogenic cells of infarcted muscle origin mistakenly known as erythrophagocytes (fig. 73)

Figure 73. This figure demonstrates the development of red cells and cells that are usually termed histiocytes or phagocytes, and a few lymphocytes from infarcted muscle fibers. (A), a barely visible group of red cells

arising from an infarcted myofiber. (B) red cells where infarcted muscle elements (the mother substance) have mostly disappeared. (C) similarly developed red cells within a capillary. (D) cells derived from infarcted myoplasm, commonly known as histiocytes or phagocytes. (E) is a cell with similar origin as (D) from which red cells are arising, such cells are commonly and mistakenly called 'erythrophagocytes' instead of erythrogenic cells. H&E x 520

Massive red cell formation directly from fresh infarcted muscle fibers with replacement of the latter (figs. 74 and 75)

Figures 74 and 75. These figures show profusely developing red cells from infarcted myofibers. In figure 74, many of these red cells are free from muscle elements. In figure 75, in the lower left diagonal area, the vanishing infarcted myofibers are packed with developing red cells. (Compare the similar development of red cells in liver parenchyma of the same patient in figure 76.) Figure 74, H&E x 520; and figure 75, H&E x 260

Markedly congested liver of the same patient showing replacement of necrosed liver cells with developing red cells causing what is known as hemorrhagic necrosis (fig. 76)

Figure 76. In the upper right segment, the dissolution of blood forming infarcted liver parenchyma is contributing to the development of blood sinusoids. In the mid area, the necrosed liver cell cords are packed with developing red cells. Lying obliquely on the left, what is probably a new central vein unit (A) is developing from the dissolving necrosed liver parenchyma with production of red cells, plasma, and lining endothelium. In the lumen of this developing blood vessel, the arrow points to the liver cells not yet completely dissolved and still producing red cells. H&E x 260

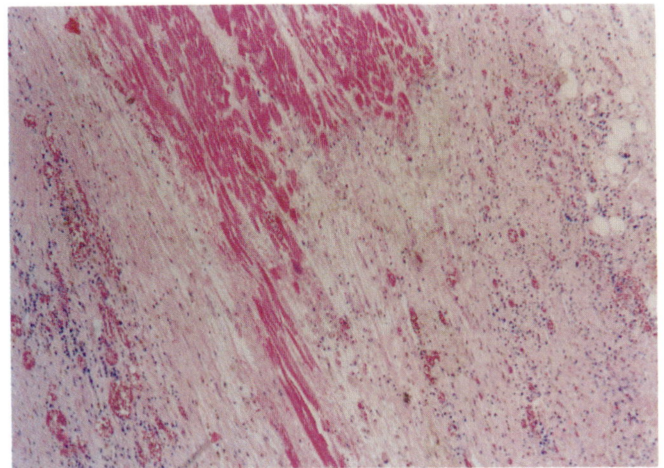

Figure 71

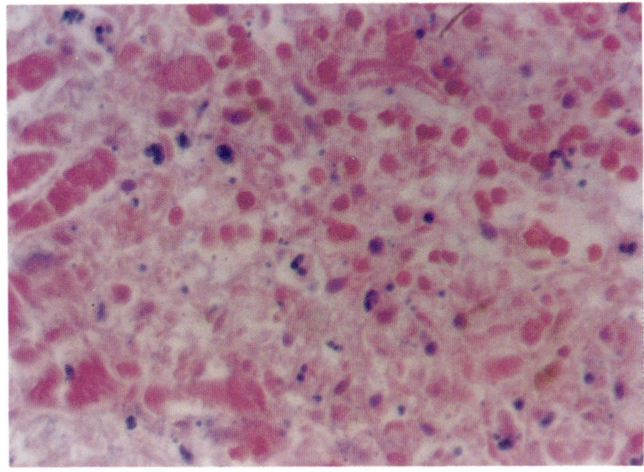

Figure 72

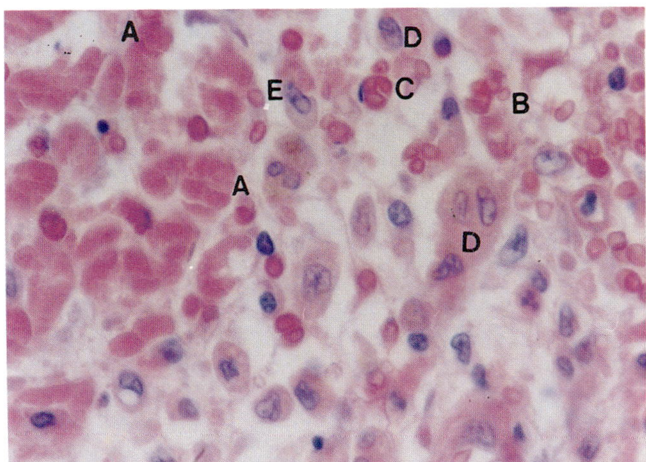

Figure 73

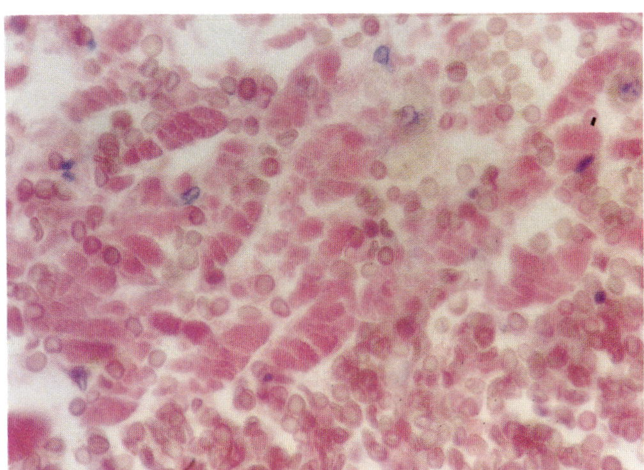

Figure 74

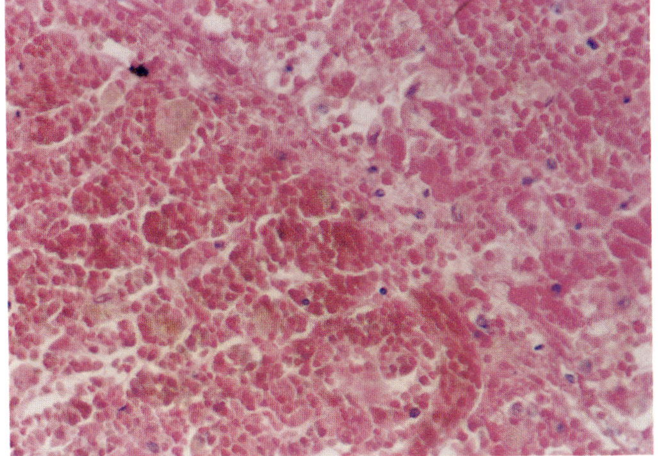

Figure 75

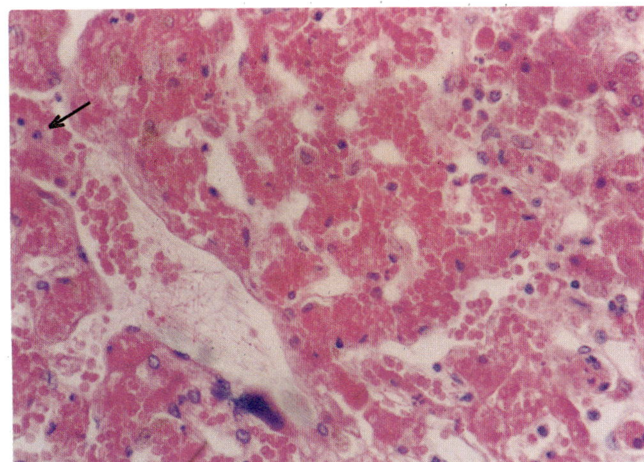

Figure 76

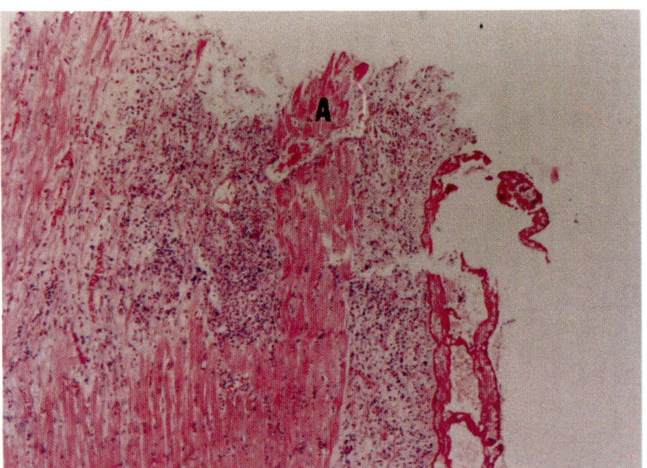

Figure 77

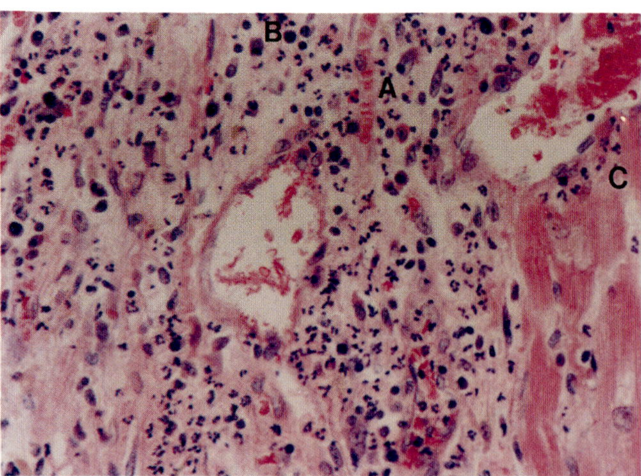

Figure 78

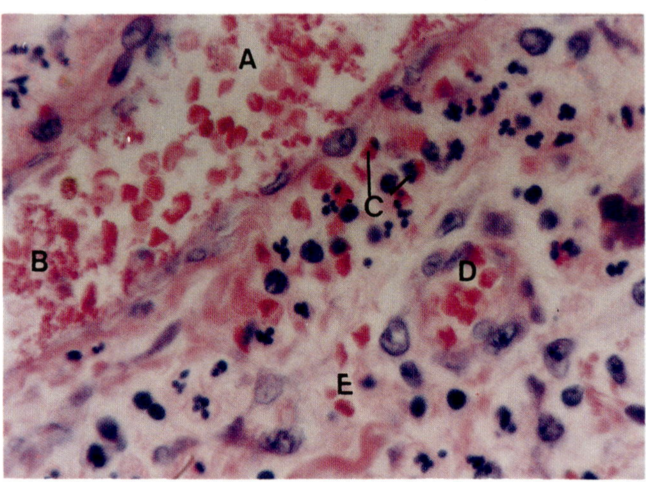

Figure 79

3. Acute regional myocarditis with outer extension as fibrinous pericarditis (figs. 77-81)

Figure 77. Proliferation of acute inflammatory cells (see next figure for higher magnification) arising from noninfarcted cardiac muscle fibers extends to the epicardial surface, on the right, where deep red hemoglobin gel-like substance covers the outer surface of the heart. On the left of (A) there is a developing blood capillary with remains of infarcted muscle element in the lumen. Note, there is evidence of infarction covering certain parts of the myofiber around (A). H&E x 52

Development of acute inflammatory cells— mainly segmented nuclear cells (SN cells like those of suppurative inflammation)—and blood capillaries from disappearing myofibers (figs. 78-79)

Figure 78. In this figure there is marked proliferation of acute inflammatory cells, mostly segmented nuclear cells, a few colonies of developing plasma cells, and some unclassified reactive cells arising from and replacing most of the cardiac muscle, except for a segment of myofibers on the right side. Also shown in this figure are two large developing blood capillaries arising from liquefied muscle fibers; the shredded remnants of the latter are still visible within the capillary lumen together with the developing red cells. Note that there are no segmented nuclear cells in the lumen. The endothelial lining has barely developed. (A) points to a developing capillary with a single column of pressed-biscuit-like red cells which have not yet fully formed. (B) shows a group of plasma cells of various sizes developing from hyalinized muscle fibers. On the right side near (C), SN cells are arising as minute nuclear particles from noninfarcted muscle fibers. H&E x 260

Figure 79. Lying obliquely is a large blood vessel developing from dissolved muscle fibers which are forming red cells. This blood vessel is in a further developed stage compared to the blood vessels shown in figure 78. Some red cells (A) have not yet acquired a regular shape and are less hemoglobinized. (B) points to hemoglobinized fragments and granules progressing towards their development into red cells. Parallel to this vascular channel is an ill-defined column of developing erythrogenic segmented nuclear cells with deeply basophilic lobulated nuclear structures; (C) points to these cells showing development of hemoglobin globules often clumped together in the beginning and of irregular sizes. Red cells are developing starting as hyalin globules within the formative capillary (D). (E) represents a few clumped red cells derived from erythrogenic SN cells. H&E x 520

Extension of acute myocardial inflammation to visceral pericardium (figs. 80-81)

Figure 80. This figure demonstrates acute inflammation extending to the surface where it is directly covered with an inner deep purplish-red irregular layer of hemoglobin gel

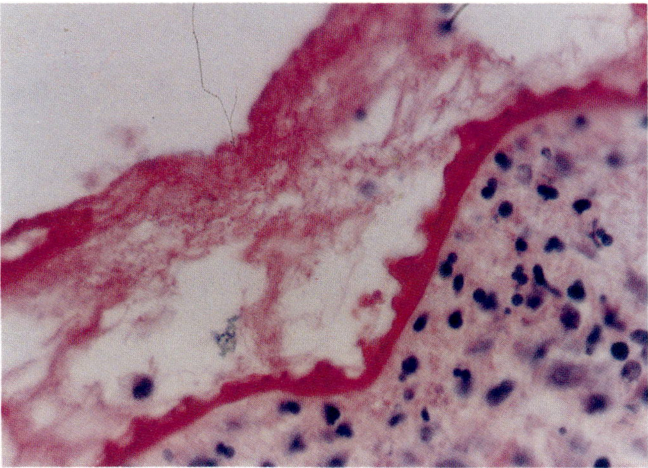

Figure 80

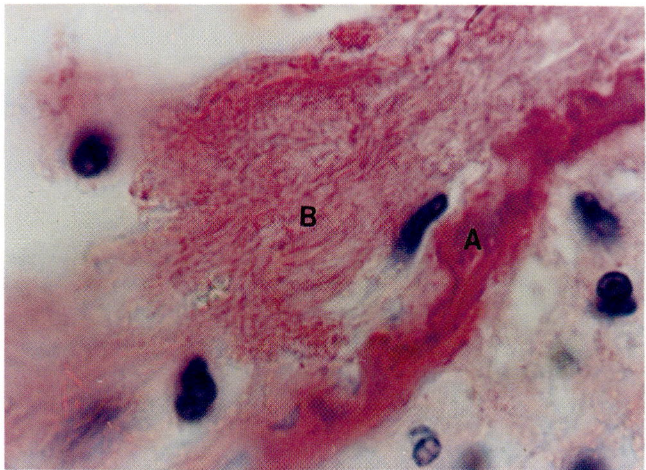

Figure 81

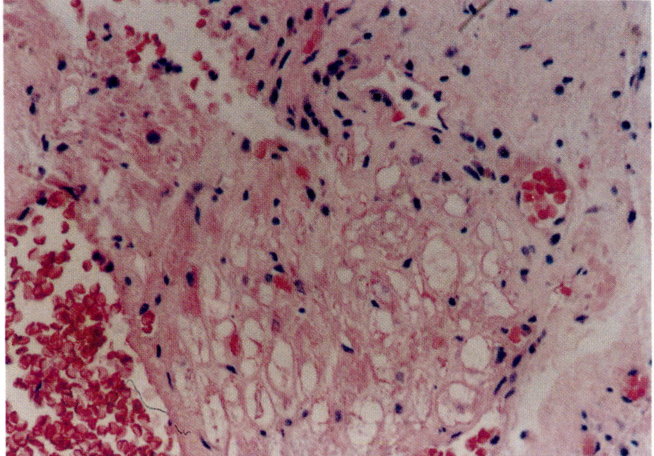

Figure 82

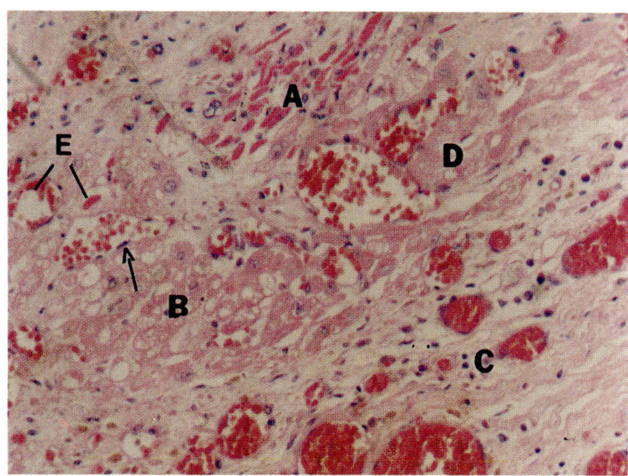

Figure 83

(see fig. 13) partially covered with loose fibrin-like mesh. H&E x 520

Figure 81. This is a magnified view of a similar area of epicardial surface close to that shown in figure 80. On careful examination, it may be noticed that the deposited purplish substance is not fibrin but hemoglobin gel-like substance (A) formed by liquefaction of the outer layer of muscle. (Development of hemoglobin gel from cardiac muscle was shown earlier in figure 13.) In the outer area (B), the red parallel fibrillary structures could be fringed and disintegrated myofibrils. H&E x 1300

4. Coronary occlusion may be associated with a variety of other changes (figs. 82-90) in addition to coagulation necrosis and acute regional myocarditis with fibrinous pericarditis

Vacuolar necrosis (fig. 82) and vacuolar degeneration of cardiac muscle (figs. 83-84)

Figure 82. Vacuolar necrosis is shown by aseptic necrosis of cardiac muscle with com-

plete erasure of muscle structure replaced by friable material with swiss cheese like vacuole formation and liquefaction. Development of blood from such muscle product is shown in this figure. H&E x 260

Figure 83. Vacuolar degeneration (close to myocardial infarction) associated with various changes in myocardium is shown in this figure. Patchy red infarcted muscle fibers are seen mostly in area (A), and vacuolar degeneration of cardiac muscle in different degrees in area (B). In the right lower region, many large and small blood capillaries (C)— packed with developing red cells—are arising from ischemic cardiac muscle which has already changed to loose fibrillary substance. Blood vessels are also developing from identifiable myofibers (D). (E) suggests stages of development of new capillaries from dissolving infarcted myofibers, the remnants of which are still present in the lumens. An arrow points to endothelial cells developing from peripheral myoplasm. (A magnifying glass would be helpful to recognize the formative stages of red cells and endothelium.) H&E x 130

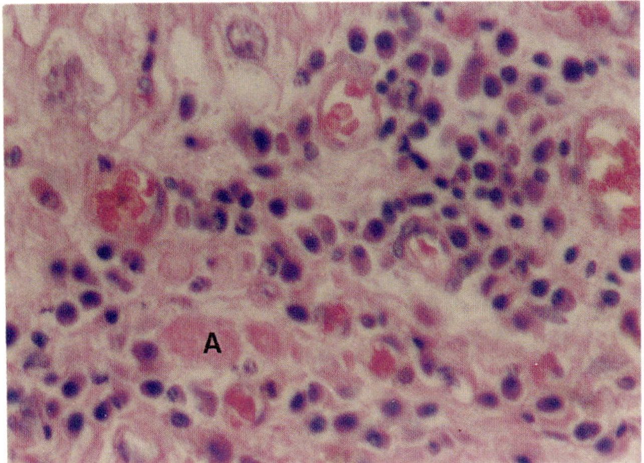

Figure 84

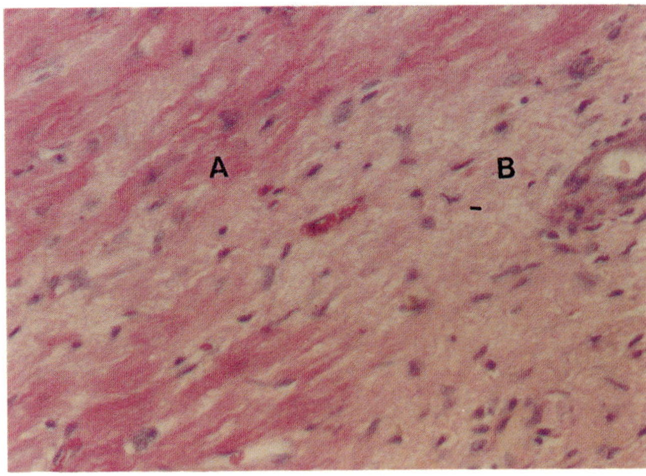

Figure 85

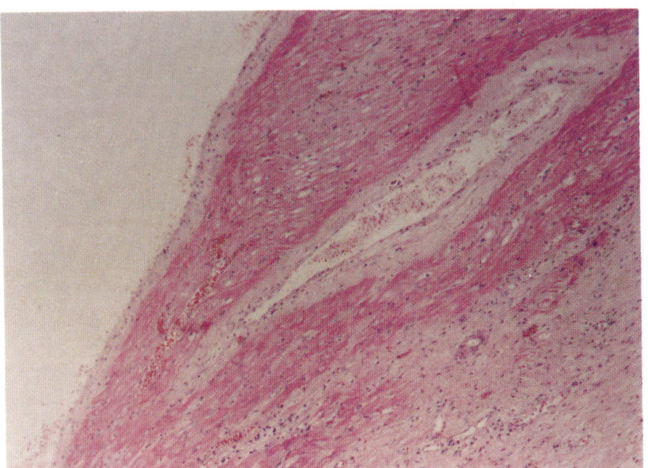

Figure 86

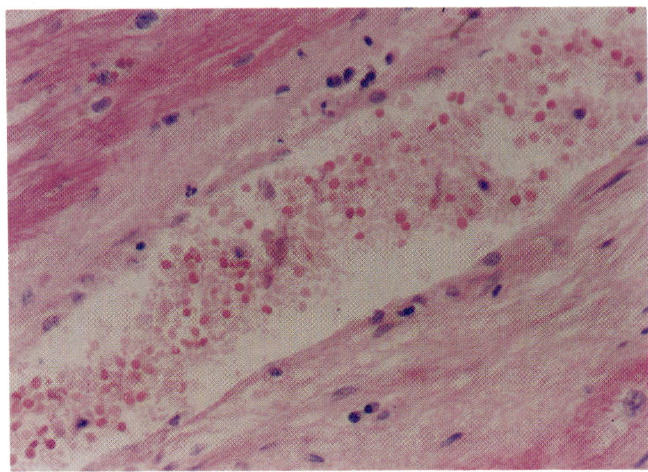

Figure 87

Figure 84. In this figure there is a proliferation of erythrogenic plasma cells and blood capillaries from myofibers with vacuolar degeneration and also from infarcted myofibers. Remnants of infarcted myofibers are shown by (A). H&E x 520

Possible transformation of ischemic cardiac muscle (in sub-optimal coagulation necrosis) directly into collagenous tissue (fig. 85); and also into large blood vessels (figs. 86 and 87)

Figure 85. The direct transformation of ischemic cardiac muscle into spindle-shaped narrow nuclei in a somewhat washed-out collagenous background (A), possibly towards development of collagenous fibrous tissue, is shown in this figure. Here instead of the initial coagulation necrosis (as seen in figure 56) the cardiac muscle fibers pass through initial changes of red loose fibrillary structures with development of narrow spindle-shaped nuclei (B), while the regular cardiac muscle nuclei have already disappeared. (See chapter two for various ways of fibrous tissue development from cardiac muscle in chronic ischemic conditions. Also see various ways of blood vessel formation from cardiac muscle in chapter one.) H&E x 130

Figures 86 and 87. In lower magnification (fig. 86), upon casual observation this large blood vessel may appear to be well established. However, in higher magnification (fig. 87) the developing status of both the vascular content and the vessel wall will be evident. Within the lumen, red cells are shown in various stages of development, from fine light pink granular undissolved element to fully formed red cells. Also the endothelium has not yet fully developed and the apparently thick wall has been formed of loose fibrillary structures derived from ischemic muscle. The mechanism of blood vessel development in ischemic cardiac muscle, as shown here, possibly explains the developmental processes of collateral circulation following coronary occlusion. Figure 86, H&E x 52; and figure 87, H&E x 260

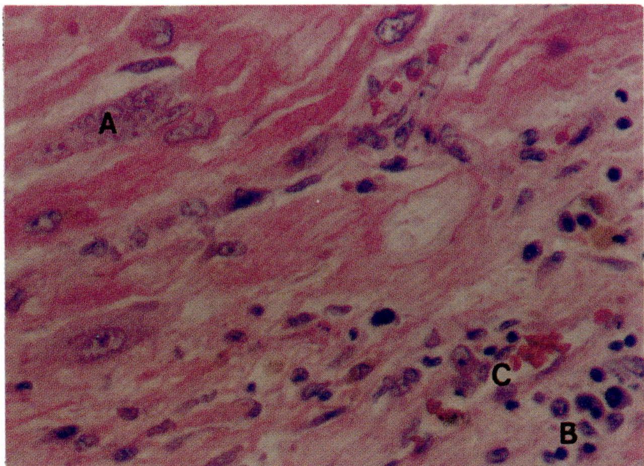

Figure 88

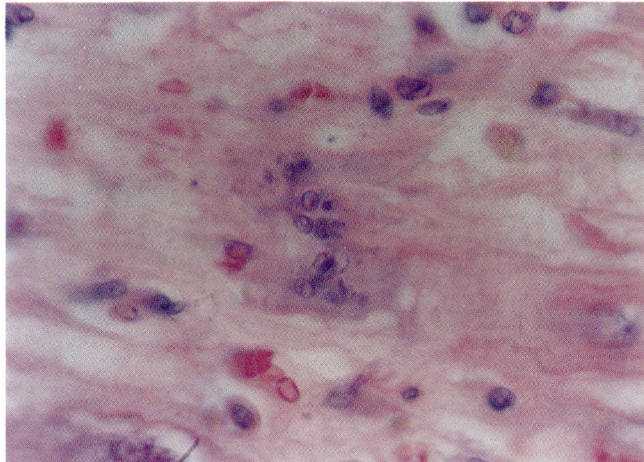

Figure 89

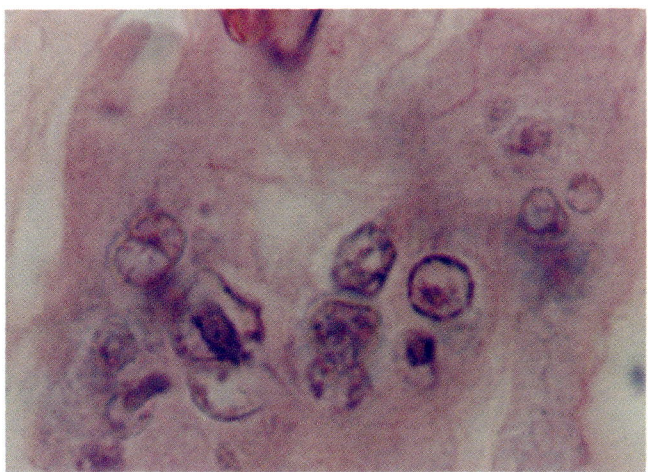

Figure 90

Ischemic cardiac muscle giving rise to atypical nuclear proliferation with formation of multinucleated giant cells like tumor giant cells (figs. 88) or fioreign body giant cells (figs. 89-90)

Figure 88. In this figure there is the appearance of atypical nuclei in ischemic myofibers from which cross striations and regular nuclei have already disappeared. There are many large nuclei clumped together within the damaged muscle fiber (A); this is commonly called a muscle giant cell. In the lower right there is a proliferation of reactive cells ranging from tiny cellular structures, in which nuclei are hard to distinguish from the deeply stained cytoplasm, to regular sized plasma cells (B). These tiny cellular structures, "plasma cell bodies" (first named by Patterson 1986) which are found by the author to be one of the early developmental stages of plasma cells arising from local tissue (McDonald 1989, p. 30). Also, enclosing such reactive and erythrogenic plasma cells there arises a blood capillary (C). H&E x 260

Figure 89 and 90. Ischemic cardiac muscle showing proliferation of nuclei like those of foreign body giant cells is seen in foreign body reactions. Origin of multiple separate nuclei are seen within the hyalinized smokey altered myoplasm. In higher magnification (figure 90,) one may see that from hyalinized myoplasm there is gradual development of nuclei from an almost invisible state to well-recognized hyperchromatic unclassified atypical nuclei of different sizes. Note in the mid-right section of figure 89, there are a few red cells arising from hyalinized muscle. Figure 89, H&E x 260; and figure 90, H&E x 2000

GLOSSARY

Acellular protoplasmic membrane in production of endothelium—Membranous projections derived from and passing through cellular, acellular, and even liquefied cell product at the periphery of the formative vascular lumen. This membrane outlines the future endothelium formation and supports the growth of endothelial nuclei. (figs. 1, 2 and 37)

Acute rheumatic fever—Primarily occurring during childhood, a febrile disease which is believed to occur as a delayed sequel to streptococcal infection of the throat. The exact etiology of the disease is still unknown; it is characterized mainly by its effect on the heart and joints. The most serious implication of this disease is the damage to the cardiac muscle and cardiac valves.

Anitschkow myocytes—Cells with a peculiar nuclear structure showing a serrated bar of chromatin in the center surrounded by clear nucleoplasm. These cells are usually present in Aschoff nodules in cardiac muscle and commonly believed to be connective tissue cells. Their origin from muscle fibers is shown by the author and also by Anitschkow (1913) for whom they are named (McDonald 1963a). (figs. 1, 2 and 37)

Aschoff bodies or Aschoff nodules—The diagnostic feature of rheumatic fever as it appears in cardiac muscle. Aschoff bodies consist of a variety of cells, including Anitschkow myocytes, Aschoff cells, and fibrinoid material. (figs. 26-29, 40, and 42-45)

Aschoff cells—Cells with specific characteristics taking part in the formation of Aschoff nodules which are the diagnostic feature of rheumatic fever and commonly believed to be of connective tissue origin. The origin of three types of Aschoff cells (A, B, and C) from cardiac muscle fibers through three respective cytogenesis pathways has been demonstrated by the author (McDonald, 1963a, 1975a & 1978). (Type A: figs. 26, & 30-33; Type B: figs. 35, 36, 38, & 42; Type C: figs. 28-29, & 35) *Cf. Aschoff bodies*

Aschoff nodules—*see Aschoff bodies*

Cardiac hypertrophy—Increased muscle mass usually believed to be due to the enlargement of individual muscle fibers. (fig. 58) Because of the absence of mitosis, the development of new muscle fibers is not considered to be the cause of increased muscle mass. *Cf. Regeneration of cardiac muscle fibers*

Cardiac rupture—In acute myocardial infarction, the cardiac muscle wall may occasionally rupture with profuse hemorrhage. This study suggests that the initial hemorrhage is caused by the production of blood of infarcted cardiac muscle origin (figs. 74 and 75). Also rupture may occur by the liquefaction of acutely inflamed (suppurative) muscle (figs. 77 and 78) which may be called inflammatory necrosis.

Coagulation necrosis—A type commonly produced by cutting off blood supply, i.e., in infarction, and is characterized by a protoplasmic coagulative process. In such necrosis, general architectural features may be preserved for a considerable period, although cellular detail is lost. Necrotic tissue tends to stain diffusely with red acid dyes such as eosin with lack of any blue or hematoxylin staining material. (figs. 56 and 58)

Dedifferentiation—The process by which cells return to their primitive or undifferentiated cell stages (as seen in fig. 35 and 36 from cardiac muscle). The reverse of the differentiation process, the dedifferentiated cells may redifferentiate into the same kind of cell (cardiac muscle figs. 40 and 47) or into another distinctive cell type such as collagenous fibrous tissue. (figs. 25 and 46) *Cf. Differentiation*

Degeneration—Cellular alterations with or without erasure of the local cells. The specific degeneration is named according to the morphological change or the nature of the abnormally accumulated material such as in hyalin degeneration, hydropic degeneration, fatty change, amyloid deposition, or amyloidosis, etc.

Differentiation—The process of acquiring distinctive individual cellular characteristics from an undifferentiated or primitive stage, such as occurs in the cells and tissues of the embryo, or from a transformed primitive stage reverted from once well-developed tissue. *Cf. Dedifferentiation*

Edema—The presence of an abnormally large amount of fluid (edema fluid) in the tissue. In acute rheumatic fever, liquefaction of cardiac muscle causes clefts and sinuses filled with clear edema fluid. When surrounded by endothelial membrane the fluid is called lymph and the channel is termed lymphatic channel. (figs. 36, 36 and 36-1)

Embolus—Within the vascular lumen, a blood clot or other plug brought by the blood current from a distant vessel.

Erythrocytes—A synonym for red cells or red blood cells. *Cf. Erythrogenesis*

Erythrogenesis—The development of red cells. The common belief is that red cells can only develop through the nucleated phases of erythropoiesis and only in the bone marrow in adults. The author's research in agreement with many early workers (see references) has demonstrated various other ways of red cell formation from practically all tissues, benign and malignant, and from various reactive or inflammatory cells (McDonald 1989). Specifically shown in this volume is the direct development of red cells as hemoglobin globules from cardiac muscle fibers—adult, embryonic, and tissue culture. See chapter one.

Erythrogenic gel—A liquefied red-shaded cell product as seen in H&E stain. Red cells usually appear in this fluid as if by crystallization. Commonly seen in bone marrow and in malignant tissues (McDonald 1989).

Erythrogenic inflammatory cells—Inflammatory cells with the capacity for production of hemoglobin globules (red cells). Erythrogenic capacity of segmented nuclear cells (SN cells), monocytes/ histiocytes, lymphocytes, plasma cells, or even so-called erythrophagocytes are all presented in this book and the previous volume(McDonald 1989). (figs. 6, 11-3, 67, 73, 79 and 88)

Erythrophagocytosis—A term usually given for explanation of red cells being inside other cells. The present study indicates that the red cells are usually forming there (erythrogenesis) instead of being phagocytized (engulfed). *Cf. Erythrogenesis, Erythrogenic inflammatory cells*

Fatty infiltration of cardiac muscle—Presence of adipose or adipose-like cells in the cardiac muscle. Instead of infiltration by adipose cells, it is found that these cells are actually formed from cardiac muscle. The initial finding is lysis of individual muscle fibers with the retention of sarcolemma (myocytolysis). (figs. 47 and 48)

Fibrinoid degeneration—Usually seen in rheumatic fever, degeneration of cardiac muscle fibers producing substances simulating degenerated fibrin, often homogenized with pink or red color in H&E stain. (figs. 23, 26, 28, 49 and 50). The regenerating myoplasm may also appear as fibrinoid substances within Aschoff bodies. (fig. 27)

Fibrinoid substance—The product of fibrinoid degeneration of cardiac muscle. *Cf. Fibrinoid degeneration*

Ghost red cells—Red cells of regular size and shape with a well-defined cell membrane and practically no hemoglobin. These cells are often seen in an early stages of direct red cell development. (figs. 1 and 2)

Hemorrhage—Commonly defined as the escape of blood from blood vessels, this term is usually used whenever red cells are seen outside the vascular lumen. However, when there is no evidence for vascular injury, as commonly is the case, the possible leakage in the vascular wall is an explanation given to this occurence. Erythrogenesis from local tissues is often mistaken for hemorrhage. (figs. 11-2, 74 and 75)

Hemorrhagic necrosis—A common term for the presence of blood (red cells) in the necrosed tissue. The development of red cells through the process of necrosis of local tissues is often mistaken for hemorrhage. (figs. 74 and 75)

Hyalinization—Erasure of background cellular structures often with a ground glass effect.

Inclusion bodies—Any round, oval, or irregularly shaped bodies which are found within the cells. One may compare the intracellular origin of red cells as presented here with that of inclusion bodies or secretory globules.

Inflammatory cells—*see Reactive cells*

Inflammatory necrosis—Necrosis of tissue associated with acute inflammatory reaction.

Lymph and Lymphatic channel—*see Reactive cells*

Lymphocytoid cell—A cell which has some characteristics of a lymphocyte but is not typical. *Cf. Plasmacytoid cell*

Mitral commisurotomy—A surgical procedure to enlarge the mitral valve passageway in patients with mitral stenosis (a condition which is usually caused by chronic rheumatic fever).

Myocytolysis—lysis of individual muscle fibers with retention of sarcolemma (usually seen in subepicardial myocardium). Regeneration of cardiac muscle from myocytolysis. (figs. 47 and 48)

Necrosis—The sum of the morphological changes indicative of cell death. It may affect a group of cells or part of a structure of an organ. *Cf. Coagulation necrosis, Inflammatory necrosis*

Nucleosis—Marked focal proliferation of nuclei, intracellular or from background substance without evidence of mitosis. (figs. 89 and 90)

Phagocytosis—*see Erythrophagocytosis*

Plasma cell bodies—Tiny irregular plasma cell-like bodies having both dense cytoplasm and nuclear structure. [This name was given by Patterson (1986).] These bodies are early stages of developing plasma cells (fig. 88 and also described ealier in McDonald, 1989).

Plasmacytoid cell—A cell which has some of the characteristics of a plasma cell but is not typical.

Plasma gel—The clear and colorless liquid product of cell lysis providing tissue fluid, blood plasma and lymph plasma. The author's findings indicate that this fluid has a capacity for red cell production as well as the capability for other kinds of cell generation. *Cf. Tissue plasma gel*

Prosector—One who dissects anatomical subjects for demonstration.

Pyknosis—A loss of nuclear and cytoplasmic detail and an intense basophilia often associated with necrosis or other changes.

Reactive cells—Cells that appear in the tissues as a result of a variety of stimulations, known or unknown, or as a part of the natural growth process. Reactive cells include plasma cells, lymphocytes, segmented nuclear cells (neutrophils), eosinophils, mast cells, multinucleated giant cells, and cells with less specific features such as: monocytes, histiocytes, etc. (Synonym: inflammatory cells.)

Reactive phenomenon—The appearance of reactive cells, red cells, and endothelial cells; the proliferation of blood capillaries and lymphatic channels; and the development of collagen fibers associated with spindle shaped nuclei. This phenomenon may occur in response to known or unknown stimulations or may even be a part of the natural growth process.

Red cells—A synonym for erythrocytes, red blood corpuscles, red blood cells, or hemoglobin globules.

Redifferentiation—*see Dedifferentiation*

Regeneration of cardiac muscle fibers—Regeneration that takes place by redifferentiation of dedifferentiated (tiny lymphocyte-like or tiny spindle-shaped) cells arising from liquified muscle product.

Atypical form of regeneration may take place through Type B Aschoff cells of Aschoff body formation. *see Acute rheumatic fever*

Sarcolemma—Delicate plasma membrane which invests every striated muscle fiber.

Sarcoplasm—Striated myoplasm of cardiac and skeletal muscle cells.

Satellite cells—Same as dedifferentiated cells arising from lysing cardiac muscle fibers and having the potential for redifferentiation into cardiac muscle fibers or collagenous fibers, as described by the author (McDonald 1957, 1975, and in this volume). Since these tiny cells with hyperchromatic nuclei are seen more at the periphery of the damaged muscle fibers (fig. 36) they were designated as "satellite cells" by Mauro (1961) and Church (1966).

Segmented nuclear cells (SN cells)—The author prefers this name particularly in the tissues instead of neutrophils or granulocytes since the structure of SN cells is different from that of the neutrophils present in the blood (even though they may originate in the same way). When they occur within the vascular lumen and are surrounded by liquid medium, the same cells become rounded and form intracellular granules.

Serous atrophy of cardiac muscle—Due to lysis of outer cardiac muscle with retention of some degree of sarcolemma. (figs. 48 and 57)

Spindle-shaped nuclei—Narrow spindle-shaped nuclei may arise from ischemic (figs. 17 and 18) and infarcted muscle fibers toward fibrosis. Tiny spindle-shaped nuclei may also arise from liquefied muscle cell product as shown in acute rheumatic fever (figs. 35 and 36) toward regeneration of muscle fibers within or outside of Aschoff bodies (figs. 40-45) or toward collagenous fibrous tissue formation (fig. 46).

Tissue plasma gel—Plasma gel in tissues. *Cf. Plasma gel*

Thrombus—A blood clot developed within the blood vessels or within the cardiac cavities.

Vacuolar degeneration—Degenerative processes producing vacuoles. (figs. 82 and 83)

REFERENCES

Agarwal, B.L. Rheumatic heart disease unabated in developing countries. *Lancet* 2: 910-911, 1981.

Al-Adnani, M.S., et al. Inappropriate production of collagen and prolyl hydoxylase by human breast cancer in vivo. *Br J Cancer* 31: 653-660, 1975.

Altschul, R. Nucleosis of skeletal muscle: its value as a biological test. *Science* 103 : 566-567, 1948.

Anitschkow, N. Experimentelle Untersuchungen über die Neubildung des Granulationsgewebes im Herzmuskel. *Bietr Path Anat Allg Pathol* 55 : 373-415, 1913.

Aschoff, L. The rheumatic nodules in the heart. *Ann Rheum Dis* 1 : 161-166, 1939.

Byck, P.L., Listinsky, C. M., et al. Acute congestive heart failure in a 55-year-old man. *Arch Pathol Lab Med* 114: 526-527, 1990.

Carr, R.W. Muscle-tendon attachment in the striated muscle of the fetal pig: demonstration of the sarcolemma by electric stimulation. *Amer J Anat* 49 : 1-42, 1931.

Church, J.C.T., Noronha, R.F.X., et al. Satellite cells and skeletal muscle regeneration. *Brit J Surg* 53: 638-642, 1966.

Clark, E.R., and Clark, E.L. Observations on living preformed blood vessels in the rabbit ear. *Am J Anat* 51: 49, 1932.

Congeni, B., Rizzo, C., et al. Outbreak of acute rheumatic fever in northeast Ohio. *J Pediatr* 111: 176-179, 1987.

Coombs, C. F., 1907, 1909, 1924. As reported by Gould, S.E. *Pathology of the Heart*, 2nd ed. Springfield IL: Charles C. Thomas, 1960 p. 660.

Cowdry, E.V. *Textbook of Histology*, 4th ed. Philadelphia: Lea and Febiger, 1950 p. 458.

Drummond, James. On the development of the blood and blood vessels. *Monthly J Med Sci* 19: 214 and 385, 1854. Cited by Michels 1931.

Duran-Jorda, F. Secretion of red blood corpuscles. *Nature* 159: 293-294, 1947.

---.   The eosinophil cell: studies in horse and camel. *Lancet* 2 : 451-454, 1948.

Edmondson, H.A. and Hoxie, H.J. 1942. As reported by W.A.D. Anderson. *Pathology* 2nd ed. St. Louis: C.V. Mosby, 1953 p. 483-484.

Gabella, G. and Yamey A. Synthesis of collagen by smooth muscle of the fetal pig: Demonstration of the sarcolemma by electric stimulation. *Am J Anat* 49: 1-42, 1977.

Gerber, M.A., and Markowitz, M. Rheumatic Fever, *Conn's Current Therapy*. Philidelphia: W.B. Saunders, year 1992, pp. 104-109.

Ghosh, Hemprova. see McDonald, Hemprova Ghosh.

Gould, S.E. *Pathology of the Heart*. 2nd ed. Springfield: Charles Thomas, 1960 pp. 602, 611, 612, 660.

Gross, L., and Ehrlich, J.C. Studies on the myocardial Aschoff body, 1. A descriptive classification of lesions. *Am J Path* 10: 467-488, 1934.

Heitzmann, C. Studien am Knorpel und Knochen, über die Rück und Neubildung von Blutgefäßen in Knochen und Knorpel. Wiener Mediz. Jahr Untersuchungen über das Protoplasma. *Wiener Akad Bericht* I-V: 67-68, 1872-73. Cited by Michels 1931.

Hernandez, J.A. and Steane, S.M. Erythrophagocytosis by segmented neutrophils in paroxysmal cold hemoglobinuria. *Am J Clin Path* 81: 787-789, 1984.

Horner, W.E. *Special Anatomy and Histology*. 8th ed. Philadelphia: Blanchard and Lea, 1851 pp. 37, 170.

Jones, Wharton T. The blood corpuscle considered in its different phases of development in the animal series. *Mem I-III Philosophic Transact of Royal Soc of London* II: 63, 89, 103, 1846. Cited by Michels 1931.

Jordan, H. E. The erythrocytogenic capacity of mammalian lymph nodes. *Am J Anat* 38 : 255-279, 1926.

Kaplan, Edward L. A Comeback for rheumatic fever? *Patient Care* 22:80-92, 1988.

Keasby, L. On a new form of leukocyte (Schollenleukozyt, Weill) as found in the gastric mucosa of the sheep. *Folia Haemat* 29: 155-171, 1923.

Krösing, R. Über die Rückbildung und Entwicklung der quergestreiften Muskelfasern. *Virchow's Arch Path Anat* 128: 445-484, 1892.

Latta, J. The histogenesis of the dense lymphatic tissue of the intestine (Lepus). A contribution to the knowledge of the development of lymphatic tissues and blood cell formation. *Am J Anat* 29: 159-212, 1921. Cited by Michels 1931.

Le Gross Clark, W.E. *The Tissues of the Body.* 4th ed. London: Oxford Univ. Press, 1958, pp. 181, 186, 205, 223, 250.

Lie, J.T. Myocardium as emboli in the systemic and pulmonary circulation. *Arch Pathol Lab Med* 111: 261-264, 1987.

Listinsky, C.M. Common reactive erythrophagocytosis in axillary lymph nodes. *Am J Cl Path* 90: 189-192, 1988.

Marin-Padilla, M. Erythrophagocytosis by epithelial cells of a breast carcinoma. *Cancer* 39: 1085-1089, 1977.

Mauro, A. Satellite cells of skeletal muscle fibers. *J Biophys Biochem Cytol* 9: 493-495, 1961.

Maximow, A. A., and Bloom, W. *A Textbook of Histology.* 7th ed. Philadelphia: W.B. Saunders, 1957. pp. 73, 249, 271.

McDonald, Hemprova Ghosh. Observations on the histogenesis of rheumatic lesions of the heart. (Abstract). *Am J Path* 33: 598-599, 1957.

---. The mechanisms of formation of various histologic patterns as observed in mammary tumors in mice. (Abstract) - *Am J Path* 34: 599, 1958.

---. Demonstration and significance of independently growing mammary carcinomas within the cardiac lumina in mice, with epithelial and stromal differentiation. *Brit J Cancer* 13: 115-120, 1959a.

---. Active cellular lysis, a phenomenon of growth processes and its role in the formation of different epithelial patterns as shown in mammary carcinomas in mice. *Brit J Cancer* 13: 200-207, 1959b. (*Year Book of Pathology* 1960, pp. 53-55)

---. Active cellular lysis of local tissues and transformation of peripheral remaining tissues into endothelium leading to vessel formation as shown in mammary carcinomas in mice. (Abstract) - *Proc Indian Sci Cong* Part IV: 16-17, 1961.

---. Myocardial lysis and regeneration of cardiac muscle fibers through the stages of redifferentiation of dedifferentiated cells arising from cardiac muscle fibers as shown in acute rheumatic heart disease. (Abstract) - *Anat Record* 142: 257, 1962a.

---. Evidences in favor of fibrous metaplasia of cardiac muscle fibers in cases of gradual diminution of vascular supply. (Abstract) *Anat Record* 142: 318, 1962b.

---. Cellular lysis of local tissue in the formation of vascular lumens and the peripheral remaining tissue transforming into endothelium shown in chick embryos and humans. (Abstract)- *13thAnnual Veterans Administration Medical Research Conference Program.* p, 111, 1962c.

---. Formation of new vascular channels from local tissues by cellular lysis as shown in mammary carcinomas in mice. *J Indian Med Assoc* 39: 115-123, 1962d.

---. Origin of Anitschkow's myocytes from cardiac muscle fibers. *Texas Medicine (formerly Texas State J Med)* 59: 1062-1067, 1963a.

---. Origin of Aschoff nodules from damaged cardiac muscle fibers. (Abstract) - *Texas Medicine (formerly Texas State J Med)* 59: 273, 1963b.

---. Origin of vascular channels from epithelial tissue as shown in livers. *J Am Med Women's Assoc.* 23: 545-553, 1968.

---. Mechanism of formation of various epithelial tumor patterns and possible origin of stroma including vascular channels from cancer tissue as shown in mammary carcinoma in mice. (Abstract) - *Tenth International Cancer Congress Abstracts.* p. 299, 1970a.

---. Structural changes in malignant epithelial cells suggesting stroma formation as shown in mammary carcinomas in mice. *J Am Med Women's Assoc,* 25:493-501, 1970b.

---. Myocardial lysis in acute rheumatic fever followed by regeneration of cardiac muscle and origin of Aschoff bodies. *J Clin Path* 28: 568-75, 1975a.

---. Myocardial lysis followed by regeneration of cardiac muscle and origin of Aschoff bodies as observed in acute rheumatic fever. (Abstract) - *Program of Texas Medical Association Annual Session* p.128, 1975b.

---. Tissue lysis and its significances in composition of plasma and formation of new vascular channels. (Abstract) - *Program of the Eighteenth Annual Meeting of American Society of Hematology* p.127, 1975c.

---. The mechanism of formation of various epithelial patterns and evidence in favour of transformation of malignant tissue into benign histological structures as shown in mammary carcinomas in mice. (Abstract) - *Asia Pacific Cancer Conference Abstracts,* no.188, 1981.

---. Mechanism of epithelial pattern formation & transformation of cancer tissue into vascular channels & connective tissue stroma. *Indian J Med Res* 78 (Supplement): 29-38, 1983.

---. The possible transformation of malignant tissues into benign forms as shown in mammary carcinomas in mice. (Abstract)- *Breast Cancer Research and Treatment. v. 4 : 342, 1984*

---. New concepts in origin of blood and blood vessels from local tissues. (Abstract)-*Tenth Annual Meeting of the University of Calcutta Medical Association of America, Commemorative Volume*, 1986.

---. *New Concepts in Blood Formation and Cell Generation in Malignant and Benign Tissues: Volume I.* Waco, Texas: Diagnostic and Cell Research Institute, 1989. pp. 7-111

McDonald, Hemprova Ghosh and Calkins, H. E. Degeneration of cardiac muscle followed by cell transformation, regeneration and fibrogenesis in rheumatic fever. *Exp Path* 15: 185-195, 1978.

Michels, N. A. Erythropoiesis. A critical review of the literature. *Folia Haemat International Magazin Fuer Klinische und Morphologische Blutforschung* 45: 75-128, 1931.

Murphy, G. E. Evidence that Aschoff bodies of rheumatic myocarditis develop from injured myofibers. *J Exp Med* 95: 319-32, 1952.

---. On muscle cells, Aschoff bodies, and cardiac failure in rheumatic heart disease. *Bull New York Acad Med* 35: 619-651, 1959.

Neumann, Earnest. Über die Bedeutung des Knochenmarks für die Blutbildung. *Zentralbl f d med Wiss* Nr. 44: 1868. Cited by Michels 1931.

Oppel, W.V. Ueber Veränderungen des Myocards unter der Einwirkung von Fremdkörpern, *Virchow Arch Path Anat* 164: 406-436, 1901.

Palmer, R.M., et al. The effect of intermittent changes in tension on protein and collagen synthesis in isolated rabbit muscles. *Biochem J* 198: 491-498, 1981.

Patterson, J.W. An extracellular body of plasma cell origin in inflammatory infiltrates within the dermis. *Am J Dermatopath* 8: 117-123, 1986.

Ranvier L. De développment et de l'accroissement de vaisseau sanguins. *Arch de Physiol* 6: 429-445, 1874.

Rigsdall, R.J. et al. Virus associated hemophagocytic syndrome: A benign histiocytic proliferation distinct from malignant histiocytosis. *Cancer* 44: 993-1002, 1979.

Rindfleisch, E. *Experimentalstudien zur Histologie des Blutes.* Leipzig: 1863. Cited by Michels, 1931.

Robin, L. Note sur les éléments anatomiques appelés myeloplaxes. *J de l'Anat et de Physiol.* 1: 88, 1874. Cited by Michels 1931

Rollet, L. Entwicklung und Neubildung der Blutkörperchen. In *Hermanns Handbuch der Physiologie, Bd.14*, 1862. Cited by Michels 1931.

Sabin, F. R. Studies on the origin of blood vessels and of red blood corpuscles as seen in the living blastoderm of chick during the second day of incubation. *Contrib Embryol* 9: 213-262, 1920.

Sasse, J., Von der Mark, H., et al. Origin of collagen types I, III, and V in cultures of avian skeletal muscle. *Dev Bio* 83: 79-89 , 1981 .

Schaefer, E. The intracellular development of blood corpuscles in mammals. *Mon Micr J* 11: 261, 1874.

Schleisinger, M.J. and Reiner L. Focal myocytolysis of the heart. *Am J Path* 31: 443-459, 1955.

Schmitt, F. "Cell Constitution." *Analysis of Development.* Philadelphia: W. B. Saunders, 1955 p.59.

Schwann, T. Microscopical researches into the accordance in the structures and growth of animals and plants. Translated by Henry Smith. London: Sydenham Society, 1847 pp. 39, 66, 158.

Shaver, J.R. Studies on the initiation of cleavage in the frog egg. *J Exp Zool* 122: 169-192, 1953.

Smith, A.J. On the histological behavior of the cardiac muscle in two examples of organization of myocardial infarct. *Univ of Pennsylvania Med Bull* 227-234, 1904.

Smith, F. Erythrophagocytosis in human lymph nodes. *J Path Bact* 76: 383-392, 1958.

Spiedel, C.C. Studies of living muscles: I. Growth, injury and repair of striated muscle, as revealed by prolonged observations of individual fibers in living frog tadpoles. *Am J Anat* 62: 179-235, 1938.

Tower, Sarah S. Atrophy and degeneration in skeletal muscles. *Am J Anat* 56: 1-43 ,1935.

Veasy, L. G., Weidmeier, S. E., et al. Resurgence of acute rheumatic fever in the intermountain area of the United States. *N Engl J Med* 316: 421-427, 1987.

Wald, E.R., Dashefsky, B., et al. Acute rheumatic fever in western Pennsylvania and the tristate area. *Pediatrics* 80: 371-374, 1987.

Ward, C. Observations on the diagnosis of isolated rheumatic carditis. Editorial. *Am Heart J* 91:545-550, 1976.

Weber, E. H., and Kölliker, A. Über die Bedeutung der Leber für die Bildung der Blutkörperchen der Embryonen. *Zeitschr f rat Med* 4: 160-167, 1845. Cited by Michels 1931.

Wedl, C. *Rudiments of Pathological Histology.* Translated by George Busk. Sydenham Society, London, 1853, pp. 59-61, 82, 83, 530, 610.

Weiss, Paul. Perspectives in the field of morphogenesis. *Quart Rev Biol* 25: 177-98, 1950.

Whitman, R. C., and Eastlake, A. C. Rheumatic myocarditis: A histogenic study of the type of cells of the Aschoff body. *Arch Intern Med* 26: 601-11, 1920.

Yanagisawa-Miwa, A., Uchiola, Y, et al. Salvage of Infarcted Myocardium by Angiogenic Action of Basic Fibroblast Growth Factor. *Science* 257: 1401-1403, 1992.

INDEX

Figure numbers are denoted by **bold-faced** type.

Figure numbers are denoted by **bold-faced** type.

Figure numbers are denoted by **bold-faced** type.

Figure numbers are denoted by **bold-faced** type.

NOTES

APPENDIX

The author's three previous articles on rheumatic fever are reproduced here for the convenience of the readers. The author greatly appreciates the kind permission of the editors and one co-author for reproduction (in entirety) of these articles.

Origin of Anitschkow myocytes from cardiac muscle fibers,
McDonald, H.G., *Texas State J Med* 59 : p. 1062-1067, 1963.
(pages 89-95)

Myocardial lysis in acute rheumatic fever followed by regeneration
of cardiac muscle and origin of Aschoff bodies,
McDonald, H.G., *J Clin Path* 28 : p. 568-575, 1975.
(pages 97-105)

Degeneration of cardiac muscle followed by cell transformation,
regeneration and fibrogenesis in rheumatic fever,
McDonald, H.G. and Calkins, H.E., *Exp Path* 15 : p.185-195, 1978.
(pages 107-117)

Origin of Anitschkow's Myocytes From Cardiac Muscle Fibers

HEMPROVA GHOSH McDONALD, M.D.
McKINNEY, TEXAS

*Reprinted from Texas State Journal of Medicine,
November, 1963, Vol. 59, pp. 1062-1067*

Reprinted from Texas State Journal of Medicine, November, 1963, Vol. 59, pp. 1062-1067

Origin of Anitschkow's Myocytes From Cardiac Muscle Fibers

IN A STUDY of the histogenesis of rheumatic lesions of the myocardium, the sequence of origin of Anitschkow's myocytes has been traced from cardiac muscle fibers. This opposes the current theory that the Anitschkow's myocytes arise only from the cardiac connective tissue cells.

A preliminary report of these findings together with the findings of a few other types of cells originating from degenerated or altered cardiac muscle fibers was first recorded by the author[5] in 1957. The early investigators of Anitschkow's myocyte cells believed that they arose from cardiac muscle fibers. Oppel[9] who first described these cells in 1901 called them cells of muscle origin. In 1913 Anitschkow,[1] while studying the formation of granulation tissue in the myocardium of rabbits, observed these cells. He coined the name "myocyte" since he traced the successive stages of their origin from the muscle fibers of the heart. He also noticed the formation of these myocytes from heart muscle fibers in cases of diphtherial myocarditis.[2]

In the present paper, progressive developmental changes of Anitschkow's myocytes as seen in the histologic sections of the myocardium of acute rheumatic fever cases are presented as evidence that these cells originate from cardiac muscle fibers. Anitschkow's myocytes are seen in large numbers in cases of acute rheumatic heart disease since many of these cells take part in the formation of Aschoff's nodules. Postmortem specimens of the hearts of such cases are excellent material for this study.

Material and Methods**

The hearts of 223 patients who died with a clinical and pathologic diagnosis of rheumatic heart disease from 1918 to 1956 in Barnes Hospital were examined microscopically. In addition a few more such cases from St. Louis City Hospital and Jewish Hospital, St. Louis, were available for this study. In many instances, especially in acute cases, fresh sections including serial sections were made from zenker-fixed tissue. Altered muscle elements were studied with special stains such as Mallory's phosphotungstic acid hematoxylin, Mallory's aniline blue-acid fuchsin-orange G stain, Verhoeff's elastic tissue stain and Foot's modification of Bielschowsky's method for reticulum. In addition to conventional microscopy, cells of questionable muscle origin were subjected to phase microscopy since this type of examination reveals cross striation better. In relation to this study, the non-rheumatic hearts of human embryos, newborn infants, young and older children, and adults also were studied. The hearts of different animals including mouse and chick embryos, mice, rats, guinea pigs, cats, dogs, and chickens also were examined to see whether in such hearts Anitschkow's myocytes are normally present and also to see the origin of such cells.

Observations

There were a fair number of cases found in which death occurred in the acute phase of the disease. During the study of these

---

*A partial presentation of this paper was made at the 96th Annual Session of the Texas Medical Association in 1963 and at the 54th annual meeting of the American Association of Pathologists and Bacteriologists in 1957.

**Drs. W. Stanley Hartroft and Wilbur A. Thomas, formerly of Washington University School of Medicine, St. Louis, made the autopsy material available for this study.

The author presents evidence, as shown in the formation of Aschoff's nodules in acute rheumatic fever, that Anitschkow's myocytes originate from degenerated cardiac muscle fibers.*

HEMPROVA GHOSH McDONALD, M.D.

acute cases various phases of myocardial alterations were often demonstrated in a single section giving a unique opportunity to study the process of evolution of Anitschkow's myocytes from cardiac muscle fibers. These developmental stages are shown here with photomicrographs taken from the left ventricular myocardium of three patients who died in their childhood of acute rheumatic fever which was diagnosed clinically and at necropsy. Fig. 1 and Fig. 3 are taken from a case of a nine-year-old boy who died two months after the initial cardiac symptoms. Figs. 2 and 4 are from a case of a four-year-old girl who died two and a half months after the initial cardiac symptoms. Fig. 5 is taken from a nine-year-old who died on the 26th day of hospitalization during which the diagnosis of acute rheumatic heart disease was first made.

There is no disagreement with the description of the peculiar nuclear structures of Anitschkow's myocytes as observed by the earlier and later authors. The Anitschkow's myocytes have been described as having an elliptic and vacuolated nucleus with a serrated bar of chromatin material in the center surrounded by clear nucleoplasm. In the transverse plane these nuclei are observed as round or oval forms with the dark central chromatin mass surrounded by clear nucleoplasm.

The earliest evidence of the origin of Anitschkow's myocyte is found in the structural changes in the nuclei of the cardiac muscle fibers in which cross striations may still be discernible in longitudinal planes of the muscle fibers (Fig. 1). Also evident is the close approximation of successive stages, A to E, of Anitschkow's myocyte formation from the cardiac muscle fibers. The nucleus A shows narrowing when compared with normal cardiac cell nucleus. In nucleus B there is chromatin concentration in a rod shape paralleled to the longitudinal plane of the muscle fiber. Seen in nucleus C is a chromatin bar with serrated margins and a less dense peripheral rim of nucleoplasm. In nucleus D there is a sharper nuclear boundary, a thinner chromatin bar, and a clearer peripheral nucleoplasm as compared with the two previous stages, B and C. Attached to the right end of nucleus D there is a narrow strip of cytoplasm with faintly demonstrable cross striation. This is also noted in Fig. 2 F. This attached strip of sarcoplasm might be responsible for the longitudinal pull of the nucleus; when this pull no longer is active, such as after dissolution or other kind of degeneration of the sarcoplasm, the nuclei assume an oval or elliptical shape as noted in Anitschkow's myocytes, E in Fig. 1 and E in Fig. 2. These nuclei are surrounded by liquefied sarcoplasm with a few strands of remaining fibrillary material. Many muscle fibers contain Anitschkow's myocyte nuclei instead of normal cardiac muscle nuclei. These are shown in transverse sections in Fig. 3. Cross striations which can still be detected in some of these muscle fibers on microscopic examination, are not too clear in this photomicrograph. However, sarcolemmic boundaries of these muscle fibers containing Anitschkow's myocytes are better demonstrated in transverse planes than those in the longitudinal planes of the muscle fibers. (Compare with Figs. 6 and 7.)

Degeneration or alteration of muscle fibers seems to be associated with the origin of Anitschkow's myocytes. The sarcoplasm undergoes a combination of various types of degeneration which may be seen as hyaline, fibrinoid, fibrillary, vacuolar, and liquefaction degeneration. Finally, most Anitsch-

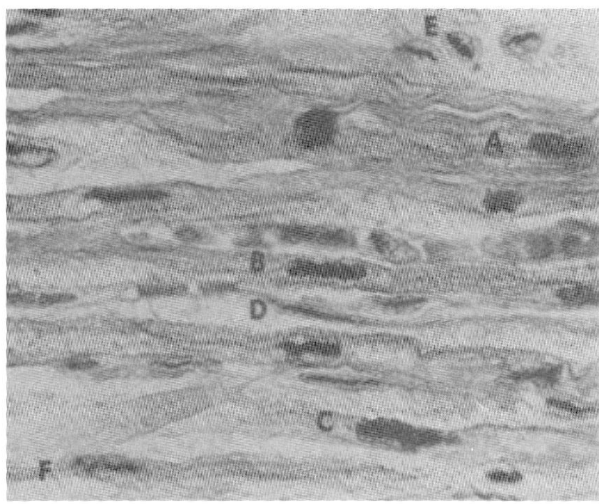

Fig. 1. Left ventricular myocardium of a nine-year-old patient who died of acute rheumatic heart disease. Successive stages of development of Anitschkow's myocytes from cardiac muscle fibers are shown in longitudinal planes of muscle bundles. Hematoxylin and eosin X 560.

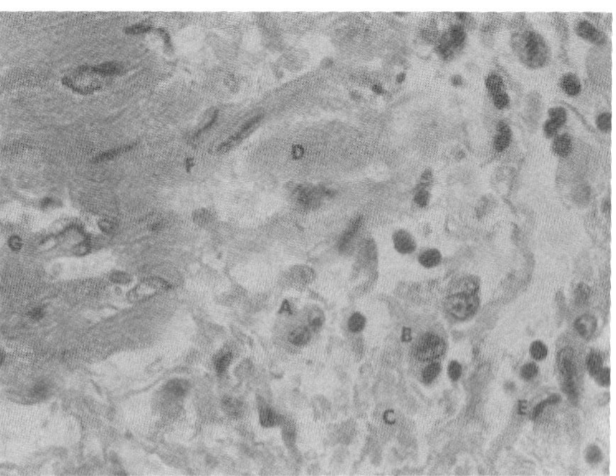

Fig. 2. Left ventricular myocardium of a four-year-old girl who died of acute rheumatic heart disease. Hyaline and fibrinoid degeneration of cardiac muscle fibers in the formation of Aschoff's nodule is shown here. Also suggested is the origin of Anitschkow's myocytes from muscle fibers and their further development into Aschoff's cells. Hematoxylin and eosin X 500.

kow's myocytes are released from the boundary of the mother cells. Sometimes a portion of degenerated sarcoplasm can be seen attached to the Anitschkow's myocyte nuclei free from the sarcolemmic boundary of the mother cells. Hyaline and fibrinoid degeneration associated with liquefaction can be seen in Fig. 3. Wavy fibrillary change of muscle fibers is noticeable in the left lower portion of Fig. 1. At the center of the same figure, vacuolar degeneration of muscle fiber can also be seen. In Fig. 4, the sarcoplasmic structure appears to be fading away in the muscle fiber *A* containing multiple Anitschkow's myocyte nuclei.

Prominent degenerative changes in the muscle with formation of what is termed fibrinoid material are demonstrated in Fig. 2, pointed out by *C*. Even in similar areas it is possible occasionally to demonstrate the presence of cross striations and staining properties characteristic of cardiac muscle. The degenerating sarcoplasm may have the appearance of fibrinoid as seen in Aschoff nodules; this becomes apparent when one examines the actively forming Aschoff nodules where muscle fibers are undergoing degeneration, and identification of cardiac muscle elements still can be made among the degenerating material. In the peripheral zone of Fig. 2, one can see disintegrating muscle giving rise to what may be called fibrinoid material. Relatively well-preserved muscle fibers such as pointed out by *D* may frequently be noticed among the disintegrated muscle fibers.

Throughout this study it is suggested that degenerated cardiac muscle fibers soon lose their characteristic staining properties and cross striations and become indistinguishable from degenerated collagenous fibrous tissue. The origin of fibrinoid material of Aschoff's nodule from cardiac muscle has been well documented by Murphy.[7, 8]

Proliferation of Anitschkow's myocytes frequently is seen in cases of acute rheumatic fever. This is obvious in Fig. 3 by *A* and *B* and in Fig. 4 by *A* where proliferation of Anitschkow's myocytes can be seen while they are still within the sarcolemmic boundary of muscle fibers. Proliferation of these cells is also seen after their release from the mother cells (Fig. 5). Mitosis is seen rarely. The nuclear configuration in the process of multiplication of Anitschkow's myocytes as pointed out by *F* in Fig. 1, *A* and *G* in Fig. 2, *A* in Fig. 3, *A* in Fig. 4, and in Fig. 5 favors the direct division or amitosis as believed by Anitschkow as a main mechanism for multiplication of these myocytes. However, the nuclear configuration of the multinucleated Anitschkow's myocytes pointed out by *B* in Fig. 3 cannot rule out the possibility of endomitosis with polyploidy.

The owl-eyed Aschoff's cell which is frequently noticed in rheumatic fever is shown in Fig. 2 by *A* and *B*. Here also the nuclear configuration of these owl-eyed Aschoff's cells suggests their formation by direct division of Anitschkow's myocytes.

Other types of cell changes in Anitschkow's myocytes were also studied. One of

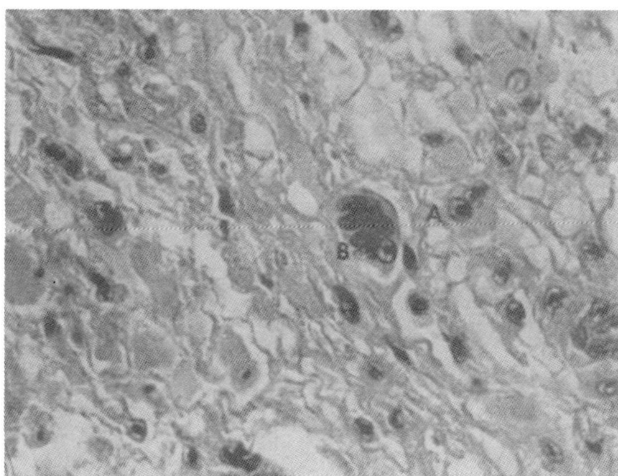

Fig. 3. Left ventricular myocardium of the same heart as shown in Fig. 1. Degenerating cardiac muscle fibers containing Anitschkow's myocyte nuclei are shown in transverse sections. Note that sarcolemmic boundaries are still present in muscle fibers containing one or more Anitschkow's myocyte nuclei. Hematoxylin and eosin X 450.

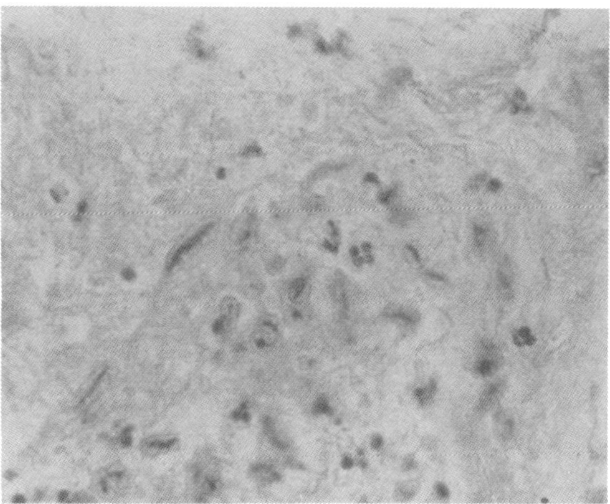

Fig. 4. Left ventricular myocardium of the same heart as shown in Fig. 2. Multiplication of Anitschkow's myocyte nuclei can be seen in the hyalinized cardiac muscle fibers as pointed out by A. Marked degeneration of muscle fibers with liquefaction observed in lower and right side of the picture. Hematoxylin and eosin X 300.

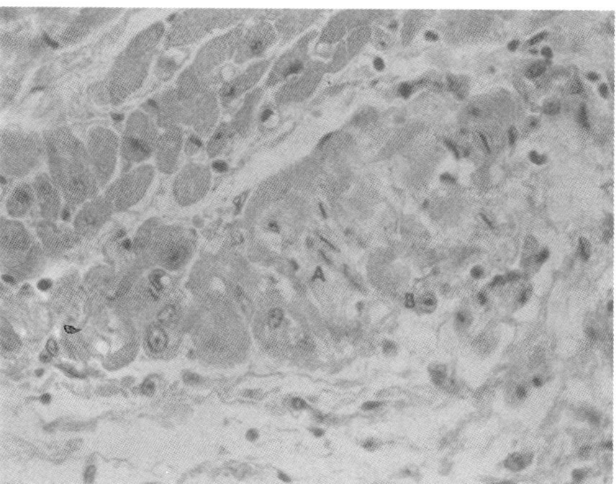

Fig. 5. Left ventricular myocardium of a nine-year-old patient who died of acute rheumatic heart disease. Highly atypical proliferation of Anitschkow's myocytes is suggested by their nuclear configuration. Also seen is the origin of cells mimicking polymorphonuclear leukocytes from Anitschkow's myocytes. Hematoxylin and eosin X 540.

these changes is shown in the myocardium of the left ventricular wall (Fig. 5) where, in addition to proliferation of Anitschkow's myocytes, proliferation of cells mimicking polymorphonuclear leukocytes from Anitschkow's myocytes can be seen. The cardiac muscle fibers as shown here are almost completely disintegrated; only a small portion of remaining muscle fibers still may be identified at the right lower border.

Since the cytoplasms of the Anitschkow's myocyte is derived from the changed myoplasm of the degenerating cardiac muscle fiber, the sarcolemmic boundary in the initial stage is the cell boundary of the Anitschkow's myocytes. Later, when the myocytes are released from the sarcolemmic boundary because of the liquefaction of muscle fibers, the margin of the adherent altered myoplasm, when present, forms new cell margins of Anitschkow's myocytes. In later stages Anitschkow's myocytes are surrounded by fibrillary collagenous material, and they take part in the formation of scars. The author agrees with Anitschkow[1] who described the prominent role of these myocytes in cicatrization of myocardium.

The presence of Anitschkow's myocytes and their origin from cardiac muscle fibers have also been verified in this study in non-rheumatic young and adult human hearts, in human embryos, and in newborn infants. The same results have been obtained in different animal species examined, such as mice, rats, guinea pigs, cats, dogs, chickens, and mouse and chick embryos.

Discussion

Evidence is presented that Anitschkow's myocytes originate from cardiac muscle fibers. The transformation of cardiac muscle nuclei into typical Anitschkow's myocyte nuclei is shown by their successive developmental stages while surrounded by the sarcolemmic boundary. Since the nuclear changes are also associated with cytoplasmic changes which may be classified under various types of degeneration, including fibrinoid degeneration, the Anitschkow's myocytes soon lose their connection with the mother

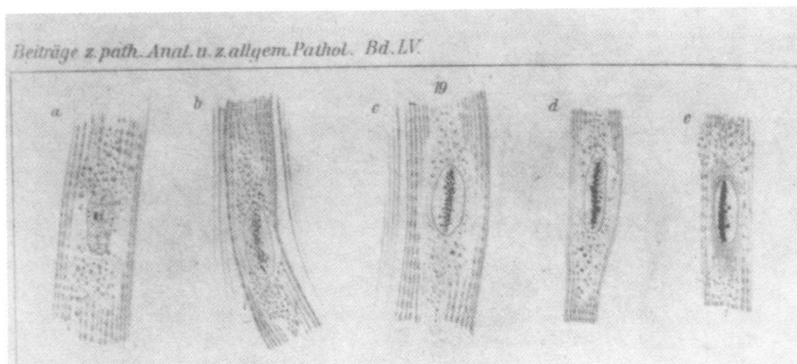

Fig. 6. Photographic reproduction of Fig. 19 from Anitschkow.[1]

cells, that is, the cardiac muscle cells. Unless one carefully studies the initial changes in the cardiac muscle fibers in the formation of Anitschkow's myocytes, it is likely that a wrong impression will be obtained regarding their site of origin since Anitschkow's myocytes will soon be seen in the material which has more apparent similarities to collagen than the muscle element. The rapid loss of cross striation together with quick disappearance of specific staining properties in the degenerating muscle fibers appears partly responsible for the origin of the current theory that Anitschkow's myocytes do not arise from cardiac muscle fibers as supported by Ehrlick and Lapan,[4] Clawson,[3] and recently by Rubenstone and Saphir.[10]

The author confirms by photomicrography the findings of Anitschkow who, by hand drawings, tried to demonstrate his findings of similar successive cellular changes in the origin of Anitschkow's myocytes from cardiac muscle fibers. The formation of such myocytes within the cardiac muscle fibers, as shown by Anitschkow in longitudinal and transverse planes, are reproduced in Figs. 6 and 7 from his article[1] published in 1913.

Regeneration of muscle from Anitschkow's myocytes has also been noticed, but much less than that of myocardial regeneration from dedifferentiated cardiac muscle cells. The latter cells have also been seen arising from degenerated or altered cardiac muscle fibers and taking part in the formation of Aschoff's nodules.[6]

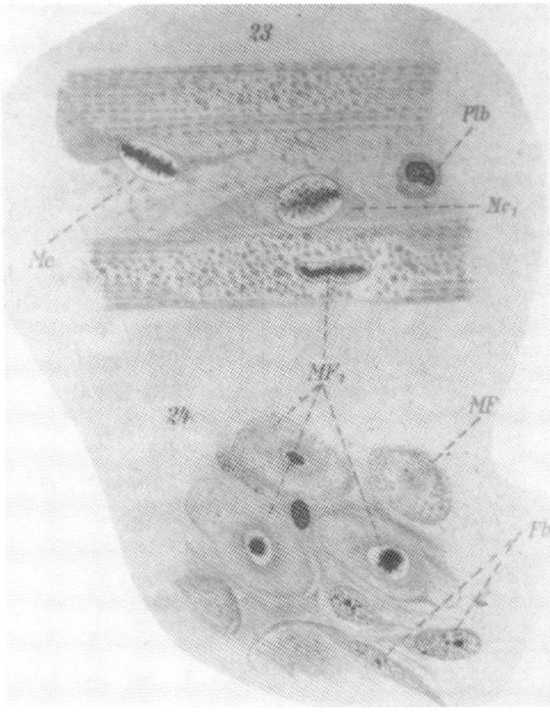

Fig. 7. Photographic reproduction of Figs. 23 and 24 from Anitschkow.[1]

Summary

The origin of Anitschkow's myocytes from cardiac muscle fibers was observed by following successive developmental stages in the histologic sections of many rheumatic hearts. This finding has also been verified in non-rheumatic hearts and in the hearts of various species of animals. The earliest evidence for the origin of Anitschkow's myocytes was found in the structural changes of the cardiac muscle cell nuclei associated with degenerative changes in the sarcoplasm. With the destruction of the sarcolemmic boundary, the Anitschkow's myocytes become released from the mother cells, that is, cardiac muscle cells. A noticeable proliferation of Anitschkow's myocytes within the sarcolemmic boundary of the muscle cells, as well as after their release from the cardiac muscle cells, has often been observed in cases of acute rheumatic fever. Mitosis in Anitschkow's myocytes is rare, whereas evidence for direct division or amitosis in multiplication

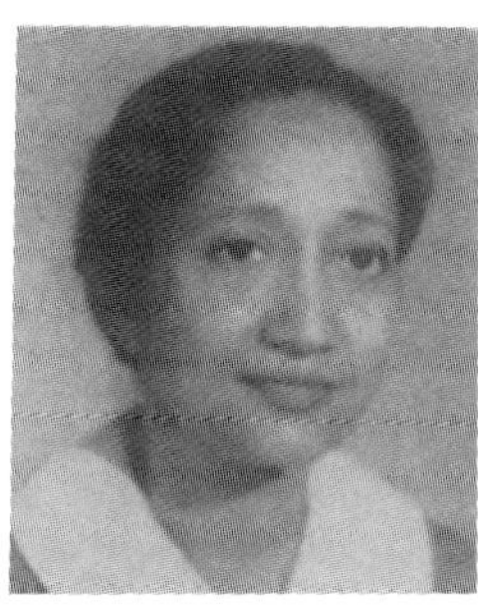

Dr. McDonald, formerly with the Department of Surgical Pathology, Washington University School of Medicine, St. Louis, is now with the Veterans Administration Hospital in McKinney, Tex.

of Anitschkow's myocytes was often noticed in this study. Degenerating muscle elements and Anitschkow's myocytes were shown to take part in the formation of Aschoff's nodules.

REFERENCES

1. Anitschkow, N.: Experimentelle Untersuchungen über die Neubildung des Granulationsgewebes im Herzmuskel, Beitr. Path. Anat. 55:373, 1913.

2. Anitschkow, N.: Über die Histogenese der Myokardveränderungen bei einigen Intoxication, Virchow Arch. Path. Anat. 211:193, 1913.

3. Clawson, B. J.: Relation of "Anitschkow Myocyte" to Rheumatic Inflammation, Arch. Path. 32:760 (Nov.) 1941.

4. Ehrlich, J. C., and Lapan, B.: Anitschkow "Myocyte," Arch. Path. 28:361 (Sept.) 1939.

5. Ghosh, H.: Observations on Histogenesis of Rheumatic Lesions of Heart, abstracted, Amer. J. Path. 33:598 (May-June) 1957.

6. McDonald, H. G.: Myocardial Lysis and Regeneration of Cardiac Muscle Fibers Through Stages of Redifferentiation of Dedifferentiated Cells Arising from Cardiac Muscle Fibers as Shown in Acute Rheumatic Heart Disease, abstracted, Anat. Rec. 142:257 (Feb.) 1962.

7. Murphy, G. E.: Evidence that Aschoff Bodies of Rheumatic Myocarditis Develop from Injured Myofibers, J. Exp. Med. 95:319 (March) 1952.

8. Murphy, G. E.: On Muscle Cells, Aschoff Bodies, and Cardiac Failure in Rheumatic Heart Disease, Bull. N.Y. Acad. Med. 35:619 (Oct.) 1959.

9. Oppel, W. V.: Ueber Veränderungen des Myocards unter der Einwirkung von Fremdkörpern, Virchow Arch. Path. Anat. 164:406, 1901.

10. Rubenstone, A. I., and Saphir, O.: Myocardial Reactions to Induced Necrosis and Foreign Bodies, with Particular Reference to Role of Anitschkow Cell, Lab. Invest. 11:791 (Oct.) 1962.

⧫ Dr. McDonald, VA Hospital, McKinney, Tex.

Myocardial lysis in acute rheumatic fever followed by regeneration of cardiac muscle and origin of Aschoff bodies

HEMPROVA GHOSH McDONALD

British Medical Association, Tavistock Square, London WC1H 9JR

J. clin. Path., 1975, **28**, 568-575

Myocardial lysis in acute rheumatic fever followed by regeneration of cardiac muscle and origin of Aschoff bodies

HEMPROVA GHOSH McDONALD

From the Diagnostic and Cell Research Institute, Waco, Texas, and Department of Surgical Pathology, Washington University School of Medicine, Saint Louis, Missouri

SYNOPSIS In acute rheumatic heart disease, lysis of cardiac muscle fibres with or without retention of sarcolemma is found to be the most damaging feature in many cases. In deeper myocardium the cellular lysis often forms anastomosing clefts or sinus-like spaces between surviving muscle bundles, and in the outer portion of myocardium cellular lysis may leave the sarcolemma more or less intact.

From lysing cardiac muscle fibres there arise dedifferentiated cells with remarkable potentiality for regeneration. For the origin of these dedifferentiated cells, which are often indistinguishable from lymphocytes, no mitosis is seen in cardiac muscle cells. The successive stages of development of muscle cells from these dedifferentiated cells within the remaining or newly formed sarcolemma have been observed in this study. This study infers that the increased number of fibrous septa, when seen, denotes the tracks of previous muscle degeneration and subsequent replacement of it with incomplete muscle regeneration and fibrous tissue formation.

In an area of muscle lysis the origin of Aschoff bodies from these dedifferentiated cells has been followed. Aschoff bodies arising in this way behave as an abortive and atypical growth of muscle fibres in a nodular fashion specific to rheumatic fever.

In the study of hearts of patients who died of acute rheumatic heart disease, degeneration as well as regeneration of myocardium is observed by following successive developmental changes as found in histological sections. In some cases myocardial lysis (liquefaction degeneration) is found to be the most prominent feature among the degenerative changes of the cardiac muscle. From lysing muscle cells, the origin of dedifferentiated cells (primitive cells in seed state) and their further development into cardiac muscle fibres will be described. Also Aschoff bodies, the diagnostic hallmark of rheumatic fever, are found to be a focal atypical growth of muscle fibres from these dedifferentiated cells.

The histological varieties of Aschoff bodies, as described by Gross and Ehrlich (1934), are believed to be related to different ways and phases of transformation of cardiac muscle cells into different types of cells including Anistchkow myocytes in the composition of Aschoff bodies (McDonald, 1957, 1962a, 1963). This paper will concentrate on myocardial lysis and the subsequent regeneration of cardiac muscle and Aschoff body formation.

Material and Method

Microscopic sections of all the hearts of patients who died at Barnes Hospital, Saint Louis, Missouri during a 38-year period with a diagnosis of rheumatic heart disease were studied. Excellent material for this study was obtained from the hearts of patients who died with acute rheumatic fever. New sections were made from such preserved heart tissue fixed in Zenker-formol solution. In addition to the routine haematoxylin and eosin stain to study the degenerative and regenerative processes, the following stains were also used in some cases: Mallory's phosphotungstic acid haematoxylin, Mallory's aniline blue-acid fuchsin-orange G, Verhoeff van Gieson stain, Masson's trichrome stain, Foot's modification of Bielschowsky's method for reticulum stain, periodic acid Schiff method of McManus, and Benhold's Congo red stain. Serial sections were also studied when necessary to obtain three-dimensional views of particular structures. Both

Received for publication 15 January 1975.

conventional and phase microscopy were used; ill-defined cross striations were better identified by phase microscopy. A large number of photomicrographs have been critically studied in the histogenesis of rheumatic fever lesions of the myocardium.

The photomicrographs shown in this paper are taken from the ventricular wall of the following three acute rheumatic fever cases:

NECROPSY 13489 (figs 1, 2, and 12)
On 11 April 1949 the fifth day of his second hospital admission, a 9-year-old boy died of acute rheumatic heart disease. Eighteen months before death he had developed joint and cardiac symptoms.

NECROPSY 6798 (figs 3-10)
A 17-year-old girl was admitted on 8 March 1937 because of swollen, inflamed ankle joints, fever of two weeks' duration, and anaemia. She died on the fourth day in hospital.

NECROPSY 5283 (fig 11)
An 11-year-old boy was admitted to hospital for the first time on 15 August 1932 with a diagnosis of acute rheumatic fever with congestive heart failure. He had two more hospital admissions before he died on 2 June 1933.

Observations

The study of acute cases of rheumatic heart disease presents demonstrable evidence that pathological changes, including the formation of Aschoff bodies of rheumatic fever, are due mainly to degeneration and reactive phenomena on the part of cardiac muscle fibres. The damage as well as repair of myocardium at their various phases is often observed in a single section and at times in a single microscopic field, giving an excellent opportunity for the study of the process of evolution. Observations presented in this paper may be divided into three broad categories: (1) damage of myocardium; (2) regeneration of cardiac muscle; and (3) origin of Aschoff bodies.

DAMAGE OF MYOCARDIUM
Of the various types of cellular changes resulting in damage of the myocardium, cellular lysis may be the most prominent feature in some cases and may involve a large portion of the cardiac muscle. Cellular lysis, although seen in scattered myocardial fibres or in isolated muscle bundles, usually forms wide anastomosing clefts or sinus-like spaces between the surviving muscle. An extreme case of such cellular lysis is shown (fig 1). Even at this low power one is able to see that some parts of the

clefts are partially filled with a large number of Aschoff bodies; some of these Aschoff bodies are confluent. The extent of this cellular lysis will be more appreciated when one compares this figure with the relatively uninvolved part of the myocardium shown in the upper two-thirds of fig 2, which was taken from a different microscopic field of the same section.

Since the edges of the cleft-like spaces formed by the surviving muscle soon become rounded off, and the cells inside the lumina are quickly liquefied once the liquefaction process has started, it is only by careful examination that one sees the evidence for lysis of cardiac muscle cells in producing these spaces obviously filled with fluid. Lysing cardiac muscle fibres with a faint sarcolemmic boundary can be seen inside the cleft in figure 4.

The lysis of cardiac muscle in the outer portion of the myocardium usually leaves the sarcolemma more or less intact, and these sarcolemmae soon assume the spheroid shape shown in figs 11 and 12. A more recent myocardial lysis with partial retention of the sarcolemma in a somewhat collapsed condition is seen in the broad mid-zone in fig 11 which is running parallel to the outer margin of the preserved myocardium. An Aschoff body can also be seen in this zone.

REGENERATION OF CARDIAC MUSCLE CELLS
Even in acute fatal cases, regeneration of muscle fibres can be followed while lysis of cardiac muscle fibres is going on in neighbouring areas. Instead of mitosis for cell proliferation or maintenance of cell population, the lysing cardiac muscle cells give rise to primitive cells (dedifferentiated cells) with remarkable potential to rededifferentiate into muscle cells with cross striations. These dedifferentiated cells in 'seed state' are seen to arise within the muscle fibres showing various degrees of lysis. These cells arise as small hyperchromatic nuclei of round, oval or spindle shape; often multiple nuclei arise in a single muscle cell (fig 3). They soon lie in eccentric positions close to the cell margin of the mother cell; the normal nuclei of the muscle fibres by this time are usually no longer present. The cytoplasm of the mother cells may show varying degrees of change, that is, minimal to apparently complete lysis. These cellular changes in the muscle fibres are shown in figures 3 and 4. The dedifferentiated cells in the early phase of cell development are almost naked of cytoplasm when they free themselves from the mother cells or when they lie within the preserved sarcolemma of the lysed mother cells.

In the process of regeneration of muscle fibres, where the original sarcolemma is no longer present,

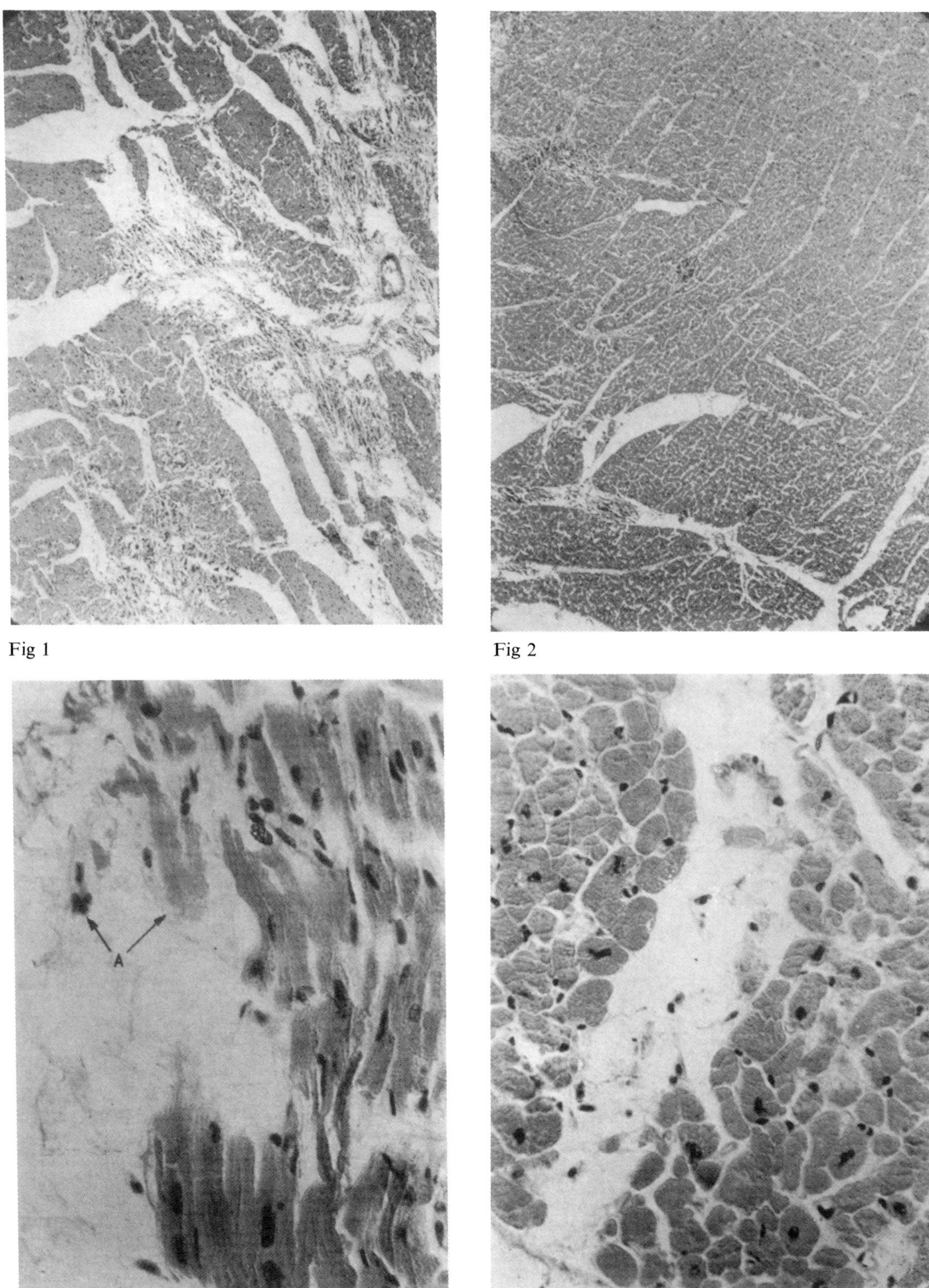

Fig 1

Fig 2

Fig 3

Fig 4

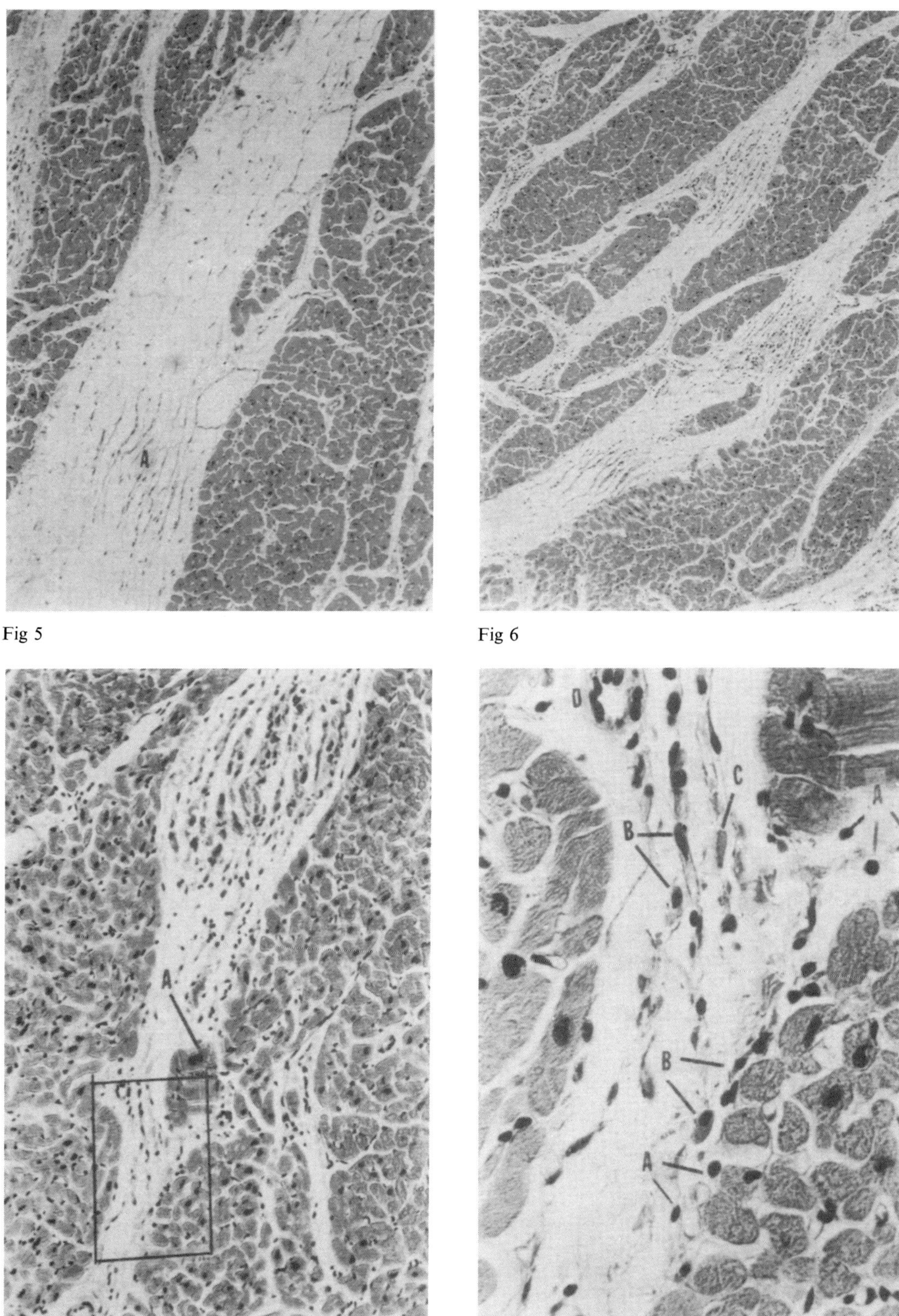

Fig 5

Fig 6

Fig 7

Fig 8

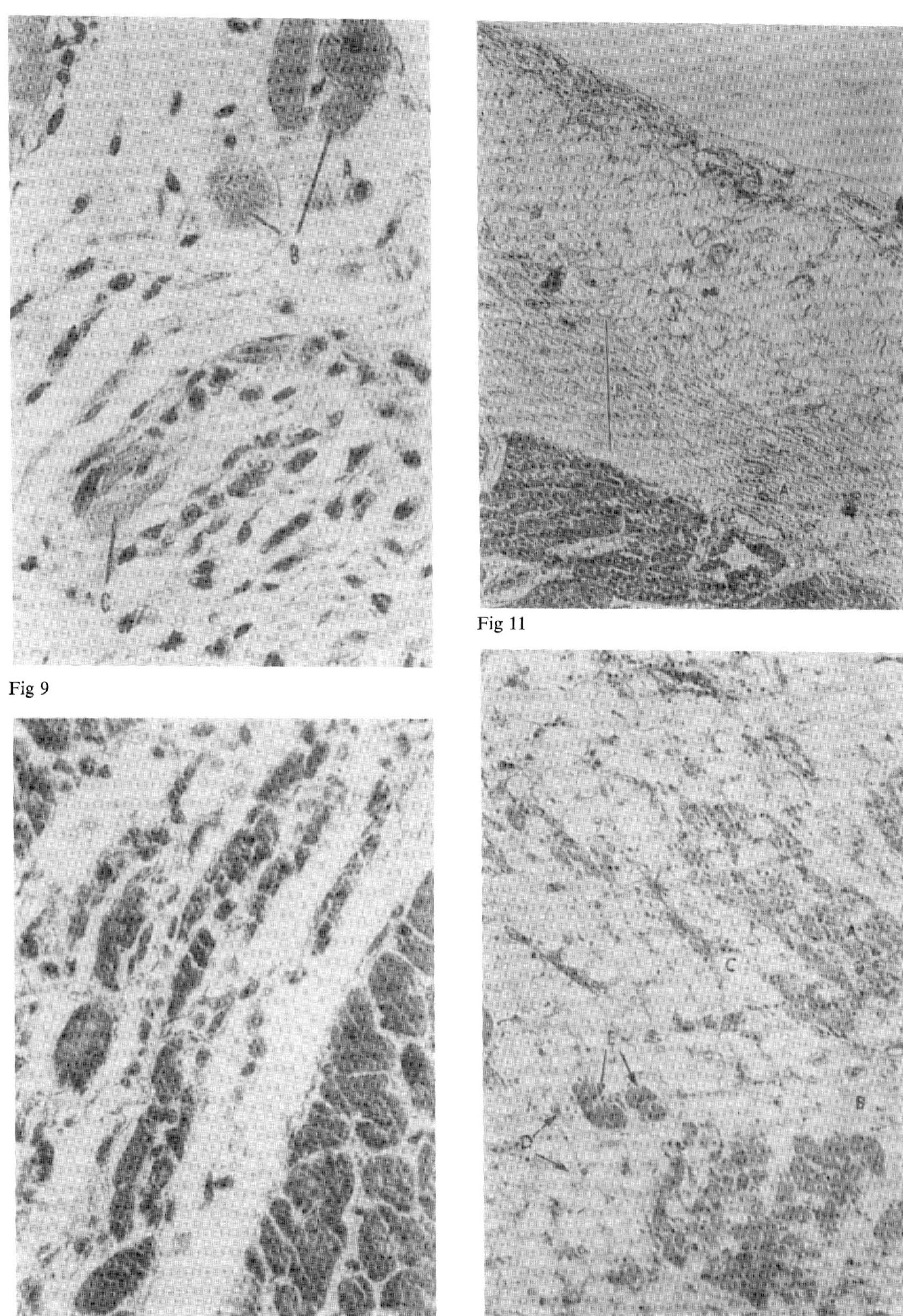

Fig 9

Fig 10

Fig 11

Fig 12

All photomicrographs are taken from ventricular walls of hearts of three patients (necropsy 5283, 6798, and 13489) who died of acute rheumatic heart disease. Figures 1, 2, and 12 are from necropsy 13489, figures 3 to 10 are from necropsy 6798, and fig 11 is from necropsy 5283.

Fig 1   *Extensive lysis of myocardium with formation of irregular clefts or sinus-like spaces and a large number of Aschoff bodies partially filling the lumina of these spaces. Haematoxylin and eosin × 40*

Fig 2   *Photomicrograph taken within 2 mm of fig 1, to give an idea of normal compactness of cardiac muscle as shown in the upper part of the field. Also demonstrates lysis of myocardium with formation of wide clefts and Aschoff bodies. H and E × 50*

Fig 3   *The myocardium near the epicardial surface is undergoing lysis. Note the origin of multiple, tiny, hyperchromatic dedifferentiated nuclei and the absence of normal cardiac muscle cell nuclei in lysing myofibres (A). Also note the disappearance of normal nuclei from many other muscle fibres. Sarcolemma of the lysed muscle cells is mostly faintly detectable here. H and E × 335*

Fig 4   *Remnants of lysing cardiac muscle fibres and dedifferentiated cells with tiny hyperchromatic nuclei and with scarcely identifiable cytoplasm are lying in the cleft-like space formed by the lysis of muscle. Note also the similar nuclei, mostly in the peripheral portion of the less damaged myofibres in other areas. Compare with fig 3 for the origin, and with figs 5 to 12 for future development of these dedifferentiated cells. H and E × 320*

Fig 5   *Preliminary stages of repair of the area of muscle lysis by dedifferentiated cells are shown. There is a delicate net-like formation by dedifferentiated cells preliminary to sarcolemma formation. A concentration of these fibrillary dedifferentiated cells in linear arrangement as the early stage of Aschoff body formation is seen in the left lower quadrant (A). Two channel-like structures lined by dedifferentiated cells in a space of previous myocardial lysis can also be seen. H and E × 78*

Fig 6   *The successive stages of spindle-shaped Aschoff body formation are seen in the spaces derived from lysis of myocardium; see also figs 7-10. H and E × 58*

Fig 7   *A spindle-shaped Aschoff body composed of Aschoff cells with shaggy cytoplasm, giving the appearance of what is known as fibrinoid, is shown in the upper part. The origin of cardiac muscle with cross striation as further development from this stage is shown in figs 9 and 10. Even in this Aschoff body under phase microscopy, cross striation is seen in a few Aschoff cells. The remaining area of the original pathway of muscle lysis becomes narrow due to the faster muscle regeneration process there, compared to the regenerative process within the Aschoff body. About an inch below the Aschoff body there is a newly formed group of muscle fibres; in one (A) of these fibres, the full differentiation of nucleus into that of cardiac muscle cells can be seen. The enclosed area is explained in fig 8. H and E × 95*

Fig 8   *Higher magnification of inset of fig 7. The same group of newly formed muscle fibres is shown in the upper left corner. (A) dedifferentiated cells; (B) myoblasts; (C) a segment of sarcoplasm with cross striation; and (D) a small capillary-like structure lined by dedifferentiated cells. H and E × 503*

Fig 9   *In the process of repair of myocardial lysis, regeneration of muscle fibres within and outside the Aschoff body is shown. (A) a myoblast; (B) newly formed myofibres outside the Aschoff body; and (C) myofibres within Aschoff body. H and E × 450*

Fig 10   *Differentiation of Aschoff cells into cardiac muscle fibres. Several muscle fibres with cross striations can be seen in this Aschoff body. Phosphotungstic acid-haematoxylin × 458*

Fig 11   *Extensive myocardial damage involving the outer portion of the ventricular wall; the outer part of this photomicrograph simulates adipose tissue but the oblique mid-zone (B) shows recent cellular lysis with partial retention of sarcolemma. In the outer and mid-zone are many dedifferentiated cells. A spindle-shaped Aschoff body formation in the mid-zone of cellular lysis is seen in the right lower quadrant (A). H and E × 49*

Fig 12   *Subepicardial myocardium showing various phases of cellular lysis of muscle fibres with retention of sarcolemma and the origin of new muscle fibres within the retained sarcolemma by redifferentiation of dedifferentiated cells. (A) muscle fibres undergoing lysis; (B) an area from which sarcoplasm has been wiped out, but faintly stained sarcolemma and a few dedifferentiated cardiac cells are present (compare (B) with fig 3); (C) an area where the sarcolemma assumes a rounded appearance; (D) myoblasts within retained sarcolemma; and (E) bundles of newly formed cardiac muscle fibres. Compare the better staining quality and form of these newly formed muscle fibres with the degenerating muscle (A) and in other areas. H and E × 49*

there appear fine fibrillary processes, many of which are connected with the dedifferentiated cells. A loose net-like structure formed by these fibrillary processes (fig 5) may act as the future sarcolemma as a preliminary need for orderly development of muscle. Regeneration of muscle fibres within the newly formed sarcolemma as further development of these dedifferentiated cells may be seen in figures 5-10. Dedifferentiated cells in the process of muscle formation are termed myoblasts (figs 8, 9, and 12).

It appears that full differentiation of cytoplasm with cross striation (sarcoplasm) is a rather sudden occurrence. Newly formed muscle fibres with cross striations stain sharply and strongly with special stains for muscle. The newly formed muscle cells within the retained sarcolemma, commonly seen in the outer myocardium, are shown in various stages of development (fig 12). Nuclear differentiation from the dedifferentiated stage to that of typical cardiac muscle nucleus appears to be almost the last stage of cellular differentiation (fig 7).

Under favourable conditions the clefts or sinuses originally formed by muscle lysis may be completely or nearly closed by the newly formed muscle; this will be better appreciated by studying figures 5-10. Less than full measure of muscle regeneration may result in the formation of fibrous septa denoting the tracks of previous muscle lysis. The potential of these dedifferentiated cells to form connective tissue elements has also been observed (McDonald, 1957). Speidel (1938), in his experiment with skeletal muscle, observed similar dedifferentiated cells arising from skeletal muscle cells with the ability to form muscle and also connective tissue elements. Church (1970) and Mauro (1961) believed that 'satellite' cells (dedifferentiated cells) arising from skeletal muscle have the potential to form muscle fibres, and Church questioned the possibility of the 'satellite' cells transforming into fibroblasts and other cells in response to injury.

ORIGIN OF ASCHOFF BODIES
While new muscle formation is going on inside newly formed sarcolemma, for some unknown reason peculiar to rheumatic fever there appear concentrations of dedifferentiated cells with fibrillary processes arranged in somewhat parallel lines in spindle pattern ('A', fig 5) as an early stage of Aschoff body formation in the space created by previous muscle lysis. In further development of this structure, one can see the successive stages of Aschoff body formation in figures 6, 7, 9, and 10. In the process of redifferentiation into cardiac muscle fibres, some of the dedifferentiated cells within Aschoff bodies acquire increasing amounts of

cytoplasm, rather shaggy with ill-defined margins. These cells, known as Aschoff cells comprising the Aschoff bodies, are found to be cells in the process of regeneration of cardiac muscle fibres in a rather atypical way (figs 7, 9, and 10). The regenerating shaggy cytoplasm, before its attainment of cross striation, has the appearance of what has been known as fibrinoid material (figs 6-10). The nuclei of the regenerating muscle fibres attain their full development as cardiac muscle cell nuclei after the cytoplasmic differentiation with cross striation is apparently complete.

Regarding the descriptive classification of Aschoff bodies into seven types by Gross and Ehrlich (1934), one can see that several of these types are nothing but the different phases of Aschoff body formation as shown here. Other types of Aschoff bodies described by them are also found to be derived from cardiac muscle fibres undergoing a variety of degenerative changes but with less prominent cellular lysis (McDonald, 1957, 1962a, 1963).

It may also be pointed out that quite frequently one may see the large or small channels lined by dedifferentiated cells, as in figs 2 and 5, in the cleft-like spaces created by muscle lysis. I have studied the possibility of vascular channels originating from these initial stages; the process has been similar to that seen in other tissues (McDonald, 1962b, 1968).

Discussion

Acute myocardial damage by cellular lysis, as has been demonstrated in this study, appears to be a direct effect of the injurious agent or a result of specific reaction associated with the rheumatic fever disease process. The loss of continuity of the heart muscle due to extensive lysis of the myocardium may explain, at least in part, the blockage in the conduction system giving rise to different types of arrhythmias.

It appears that myocardial lysis, as extensive as it is shown here, had been discarded in the past as artefact or oedema. The collection of a large amount of fluid in the myocardium without evidence of compression of adjacent muscle fibres led me to realize that replacement of the original tissue by fluid must have occurred; this process is in contrast to oedema formation in the serous cavities, lung, or areolar tissue. It is interesting to note that the experimental study of Menne, Jones, and Jones (1934) showed cellular changes (what has here been termed as lysis) of the myocardium in rabbits caused by increasing the heart rate mechanically and induced hyperthyroidism. It would be interesting to study the process of regeneration of new muscle fibres as a follow-up of their experiment.

The hopeful findings of this present study are the recognition of all-out attempts to repair the myocardial damage by regeneration of cardiac muscle. Probably myocardial regeneration has been overlooked in the past because mitosis does not appear to be the way by which the cardiac muscle normally regenerates. Mitosis in cardiac muscle has been reported in young rats in cases of experimental burn by Robledo (1956). I have not seen mitosis in normal cardiac muscle cells but have seen mitosis of Anitschkow myocytes. The process of cellular changes in the origin of Anitschkow myocytes from cardiac muscle fibres, as described by Anitschkow in 1913, has been observed (McDonald, 1963).

The dedifferentiated cells noted by Speidel (1938) in skeletal muscle and by me in cardiac muscle show the similarity of their origin and transformation into muscle fibres of respective orders. The dedifferentiated cells that Speidel found in skeletal muscle are similar to what have more recently been termed 'satellite cells' by Mauro (1961) and Church, Noronha, and Allbrook (1966) with a remarkable potential for regeneration of skeletal muscle in case of injury.

In addition, in agreement with Speidel, I observed the potential of these dedifferentiated cells to be transformed into connective tissue cells; this is seen particularly in the area of incomplete muscle replacement by formation of connective tissue septa denoting the landmark of previous myocardial lysis. The presence of unresolved Aschoff bodies along these connective tissue septa may have been interpreted as a support for mesenchymal origin of Aschoff bodies. It is worthwhile to note that Krösing (1892), after an extensive study, came to the conclusion that connective tissue may be formed as a result of retrogressive or anaplastic change in both skeletal and cardiac muscle and that this new connective tissue may form cicatrix and fat tissue.

The cardiac muscle cell origin of the Aschoff body has been demonstrated by Murphy (1952, 1959) and Whitman and Eastlake (1920); however, the extent of myocardial lysis and the remarkable potential for regeneration of cardiac muscle fibres in acute rheumatic fever have not previously been appreciated.

I express my grateful thanks to Dr Lauren V. Ackerman, formerly professor of surgical pathology, Washington University School of Medicine for his encouragement in this study, and to my husband, Dr Hendley A. McDonald, for assistance in the preparation of this manuscript.

References

Anitschkow, N. (1913). Über die Histogenese der Myokardveränderungen bei einigen Intoxikationen. *Virchow Arch. path. Anat.*, **211**, 193-237.

Church, J. C. T. (1970). Cell populations in skeletal muscle after regeneration. *J. Embryol. exp. Morph.*, **23**, 531-537.

Church, J. C. T., Noronha, R. F. X., and Allbrook, D. B. (1966). Satellite cells and skeletal muscle regeneration. *Brit. J. Surg.*, **53**, 638-642.

Ghosh, Hemprova. *See* McDonald, Hemprova Ghosh.

Gross, L. and Ehrlich, J. C. (1934). Studies on the myocardial Aschoff body. I. Descriptive classification of lesions. *Amer. J. Path.*, **10**, 467-488.

Krösing, R. (1892). Ueber die Rückbildung und Entwickelung der quergestreiften Muskelfasern. *Virchow Arch. path. Anat.*, **128**, 445-484.

McDonald, Hemprova Ghosh (1957). Observations on the histogenesis of rheumatic lesions of the heart. (Abstr.) *Amer. J. Path.*, **33**, 598-599.

McDonald, Hemprova, Ghosh (1962a). Myocardial lysis and regeneration of cardiac muscle fibers through the stages of redifferentiation of dedifferentiated cells arising from cardiac muscle fibers as shown in acute rheumatic heart disease (Abstr.). *Anat. Rec.*, **142**, 257.

McDonald, Hemprova, Ghosh (1962b). Formation of new vascular channels from local tissues by cellular lysis as shown in mammary carcinomas in mice. *J. Ind. med. Ass.*, **39**, 115-123.

McDonald, Hemprova Ghosh (1963). Origin of Anitschkow's myocytes from cardiac muscle fibers. *Texas St. J. Med.*, **59**, 1062-1067.

McDonald, Hemprova Ghosh (1968). Origin of vascular channels from epithelial tissue as shown in livers. *J. Amer. med. Wom. Ass.*, **23**, 545-553.

Mauro, A. (1961). Satellite cell of skeletal muscle fibers. *J. biophys. biochem. Cytol.*, **9**, 493-495.

Menne, F. R., Jones, O. N., and Jones, N. W. (1934). Changes in the myocardium of rabbits from augmenting the heart rate mechanicelly and from induced hyperthyroidism. *Arch. Path.*, **17**, 333-355.

Murphy, G. E. (1952). Evidence that Aschoff bodies of rheumatic myocarditis develop from injured myofibers. *J. exp. Med.*, **95**, 319-332.

Murphy, G. E. (1959). On muscle cells, Aschoff bodies, and cardiac failure in rheumatic heart disease. *Bull. N.Y. Acad. Med.*, **35**, 619-651.

Robledo, M. (1956). Myocardial regeneration in young rats. *Amer. J. Path.*, **32**, 1215-1239.

Speidel, C. C. (1938). Studies of living muscles: growth, injury, and repair of striated muscle, as revealed by prolonged observations of individual fibres in living frog tadpoles. *Amer. J. Anat.*, **62**, 179-235.

Whitman, R. C. and Eastlake, A. C. (1920). Rheumatic myocarditis: a histogenic study of the type of cells of the Aschoff body. *Arch. intern. Med.*, **26**, 601-611.

Exp. Path. Bd. **15**, S. 185—195 (1978)

The Diagnostic and Cell Research Institute, Waco, Texas, and Department of Surgical Pathology
Washington University School of Medicine, Saint Louis, Missouri
and The Department of Biology, Paul Quinn College, Waco, Texas

Degeneration of cardiac muscle followed by cell transformation, regeneration and fibrogenesis in rheumatic fever

By H. G. McDonald and H. E. Calkins

With 16 figures

(Received August 30, 1977)

Address for correspondence: H. G. McDonald, M. D., Diagnostic and Cell Research Institute, 1206 Speight Street, Waco, Texas 76706 (U.S.A.)

Key words: rheumatic fever; myocardial damages; heart muscle; Aschoff cells; Aschoff bodies; histogenesis; Anitschkow myocytes; cellular lysis; fibrogenesis; degenerative processes: myocardium; regeneration of cardiac muscle.

Summary

In acute rheumatic fever, various types of myocardial degeneration and subsequent transformation of the damaged muscle fibers into a variety of cells, classified and unclassified, are described from microscopic examination of autopsy specimens. This study suggests that in the origin of Aschoff bodies, the diagnostic feature of rheumatic fever, there are three different pathways (Types A, B and C) for cytogenesis of Aschoff cells from altered muscle fibers. Type A cytogenesis takes place through the stage of Anitschkow myocytes of cardiac muscle origin (McDonald 1963), and the Type B pathway, through the stage of dedifferentiated cells arising in lysing cardiac muscle fibers. These dedifferentiated cells with capacity for regeneration of regular cardiac muscle fibers (McDonald 1975), show abortive or atypical development of muscle cells through the Aschoff cell stage. The Type C cytogenesis of Aschoff cells takes place through direct transformation of cardiac muscle fibers which show central hyalinization of myoplasm and changes in nuclei from normal to single or multinucleated large vesicular forms.

The fibrinoid material of Aschoff bodies is shown to be the product of muscle origin. The mechanism of formation of fibrous scars in the myocardium and fibrous thickening of subendocardium are explained on the basis of fibrous transformation of cardiac muscle. Altered muscle fibers have been shown to give rise to cells which simulate inflammatory cells and others which cannot be classified.

During the course of routine microscopic examination, Aschoff bodies, the diagnostic feature of rheumatic fever, were found in a few atrial appendages surgically removed as a part of mitral commissurotomy procedures for correction of mitral stenosis in the nineteen fifties. On careful examination, it occurred that the Aschoff bodies in myocardium may have their origin in cardiac muscle as opposed to the general belief about their origin from interstitial collagen. To substantiate the validity of this impression, a thorough study was carried on utilizing the available autopsy materials from patients who died of acute rheumatic fever in Barnes Hospital, Washington University School of Medicine.

A preliminary report on histogenesis of rheumatic lesions of cardiac muscle was presented at the Fifty-fourth Annual Meeting of the American Association of Pathologists (Ghosh 1957). Since then the senior author has described the mode of formation of Anitschkow myocytes and owl eyed Aschoff cells from damaged cardiac muscle fibers (McDonald 1963). She has recently described a second mode of formation of Aschoff cells from small dedifferentiated cells arising in lysing cardiac muscle fibers and having the potential for regeneration of cardiac muscle (McDonald 1975). A third mode of formation of Aschoff cells will be demonstrated in this paper and compared with the two previously described modes of Aschoff cell formation. For the purpose of clarity in presentation, the first, second, and third modes of cytogenetic processes, as well as their respective types of Aschoff cells will be designated as Type A, Type B, and Type C.

Material and methods

The observations presented in this paper are based on the histological study of hearts of patients who died of acute rheumatic fever, in most cases before the advent of antibiotic therapy. In some cases development of the myocardial lesions was not significantly modified by the treatment; these cases afforded favorable material for the study of the histogenesis of Aschoff bodies, as lesions in different stages of development could frequently be found in the same section.

The original sections, as well as new sections made from left ventricular walls preserved in Zenker--formol solution, were used in this study. In addition to the routine haematoxylin and eosin stain to study the degenerative and regenerative processes, the following stains were also used in some, cases: Mallory's phosphotungstic acid haematoxylin, Mallory's aniline blue-acid fuchsin-orange G, Verhoeff van Gieson stain, Masson's trichrome stain, Foot's modification of Bielschowsky's method for reticulum stain, periodic acid Schiff method of McManus, and Benhold's Congo red stain. Serial sections were studied where necessary in order to obtain three-dimensional views of particular structures. Both conventional and phase microscopy were used; ill-defined cross-striations were better defined by phase microscopy. A large number of slides and photomicrographs have been critically studied in the development of our views of the histogenesis of a variety of cells found in rheumatic lesions in the myocardium.

The photomicrographs shown in this paper are of sections of left ventricular wall taken from four patients who died from rheumatic fever at Barnes Hospital, Washington University School of Medicine, St. Louis, Missouri.

Results

The extensive myocardial damage that falls into different categories of degenerative changes of muscle fibers has been observed in acute rheumatic fever. Three different cytogenetic processes, Types A, B, and C, respectively forming Aschoff cells, Types A, B, and

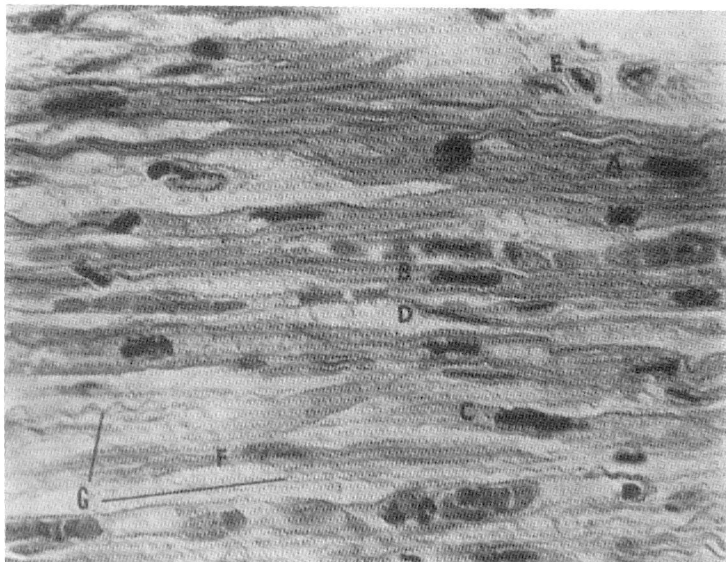

Fig. 1. Necropsy no. 5764: left ventricular wall of the heart of a 9-year-old boy admitted to the hospital on April 24, 1934 with a 2 months' history of intermittent joint pain and precordial pain for 8 days. He developed congestive heart failure and died on June 14.
Successive stages of nuclear and sarcoplasmic changes in muscle fibers, resulting in the formation of Anitschkow myocytes (A to E). The remaining strip of sarcoplasm at (D) is probably responsible for keeping a longitudinal pull on the Anitschkow myocyte nucleus. With the dissolution of the sarcoplasm, the Anitschkow myocyte nuclei assume oval form (E). A hand lens will be helpful in recognizing the fragmentation or direct division of proliferation Anitschkow myocyte nuclei (F). Compare (F) with fig. 3 (A) for further developmental processes as the dividing nuclei form mutliple Anitschkow myocytes. (G) points to wavy fibrillary changes in muscle fibers, with loss of cross striations. Compare (G) with the fibrillary degeneration shown at the peripheral part of muscle cell (A) of fig. 12, and fig. 16. HE, ×560.

C, are noticed in association with degenerations. Some other cells simulating chronic inflammatory cells and cells of unclassified nature are also seen arising from altered muscle cells. These above observations, as well as observations on regeneration of cardiac muscle within Aschoff bodies, and fibrogenesis from damaged cardiac muscle will be illustrated in this paper.

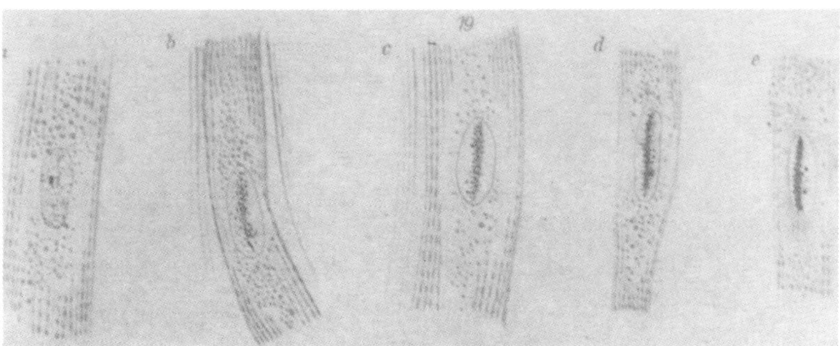

Fig. 2. Photographic reproduction of fig. 19 from ANITSCHKOW (1913), depicting successive cellular changes in cardiac muscle fibers in the formation of Anitschkow myocytes.

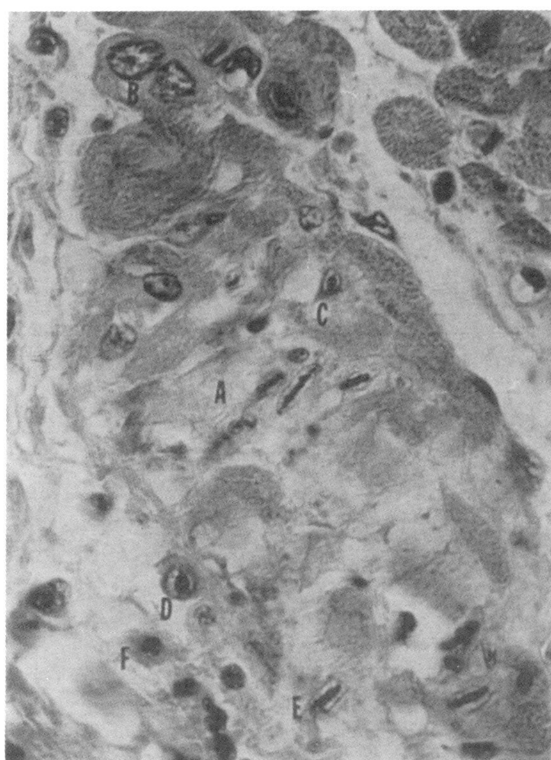

Fig. 3. Necropsy no. 8337: left ventricular wall of the heart of a 4-year-old girl who died of acute rheumatic fever on her second hospital admission on October 5, 1939. Her first admission of one month's duration was on August 2, 1939 with fever, swollen and tender joints and ankle edema. Proliferating Anitschkow myocyte nuclei in a partly hyalinized and vacuolated cardiac muscle fiber (A). (B) denotes a Type C Aschoff cell; compare this cell with figs. 11 and 12 for its origin. (C), Anitschkow myocyte nucleus in transverse section in a damaged muscle fiber. Marked degeneration of muscle fibers with liquefaction is shown in the lower and left sides of the photomicrograph, where Anitschkow myocytes are seen in transverse (D) and longitudinal (E) section. (F) denotes a dedifferentiated cell with a small hyperchromatic, round or oval nucleus arising in the lysing muscle cells. Compare this cell with similar cells evolved in the lysing muscle fibers in figs. 4, 5, and 6. HE, ×650.

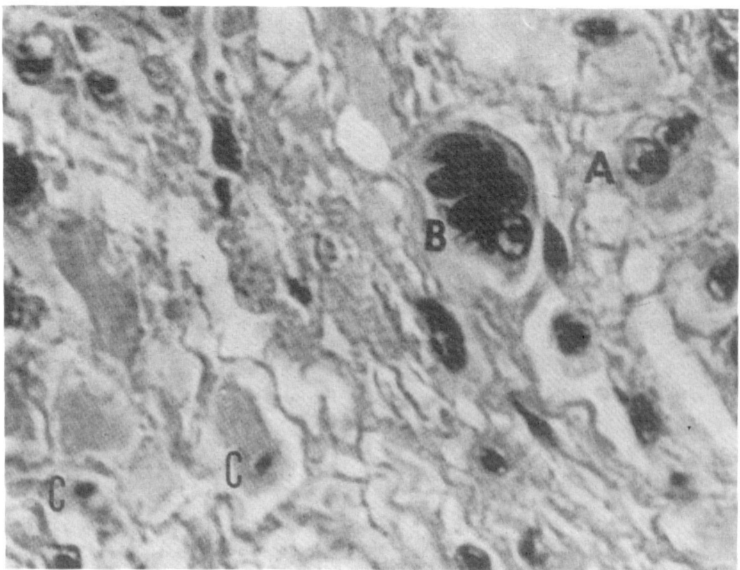

Fig. 4. Necropsy no. 5764 (see fig. 1). — Mixed degenerative changes in cardiac muscle and appearance of Type A owl eyed Aschoff cells (A) binucleated and (B) multinucleated. (C) denotes tiny hyperchromatic, dedifferentiated nuclei in the lysing muscle cell with partly retained sarcolemma. Fibrinoid material as the product of muscle damage is evident in this stage of the Aschoff body formation. HE, $\times 933$.

Fig. 5. Necropsy no. 5283: left ventricular wall of the heart of an 11-year-old boy, admitted to the hospital for the first time on August 15, 1932, with diagnosis of acute rheumatic fever with congestive heart failure. He had joint symptoms 4 months before admission. He had two more hospital admissions before he died on June 2, 1933.
Appearance of single or multiple, tiny dedifferentiated, hyperchromatic, round or spindle-shaped nuclei in lysing muscle fibers in longitudinal plane. Remnants of damaged sarcoplasm as fibrinoid can be seen in this picture. HE, $\times 370$.

Figs. 6—8. Necropsy no. 6798: left ventricular wall of the heart of a 17-year-old girl, admitted to the hospital on March 8, 1937, with swollen, inflamed ankle joints, anemia, and fever of two week's duration. She died on her 4th day in the hospital.

Fig. 6. The lysis of cardiac muscle fibers resulting in the formation of a cleft-like space shown in transverse section. Tiny, hyperchromatic, dedifferentiated nuclei of muscle cell origin, with or without adhering sarcoplasmic fragments, and with faintly visible remains of sarcolemma are noted in the space. The remaining muscle also shows deterioration. HE $\times 265$.

Fig. 7. Low magnification view of different stages in the formation of spindle-shaped Aschoff bodies believed to be in the space derived from the lysis of myocardial tissue. For detailed study of the origin of Aschoff bodies with Type B Aschoff cells from lysed muscle fibers, and regeneration of muscle fibers from dedifferentiated cells, see McDonald (1975). HE $\times 63$.

Fig. 8. Further development of an Aschoff body from the stages shown in figure 7. Here are shown Aschoff cells (Type B) with shaggy, eosinophilic cytoplasm and hyperchromatic nuclei (single or multiple) and regenerated cardiac muscle fibers from Aschoff cells. Appropriate staining methods have shown that a small amount of fibrillary material, with or without being attached to the dedifferentiated nuclei, acquire the affinity for collagen stain. HE $\times 150$.

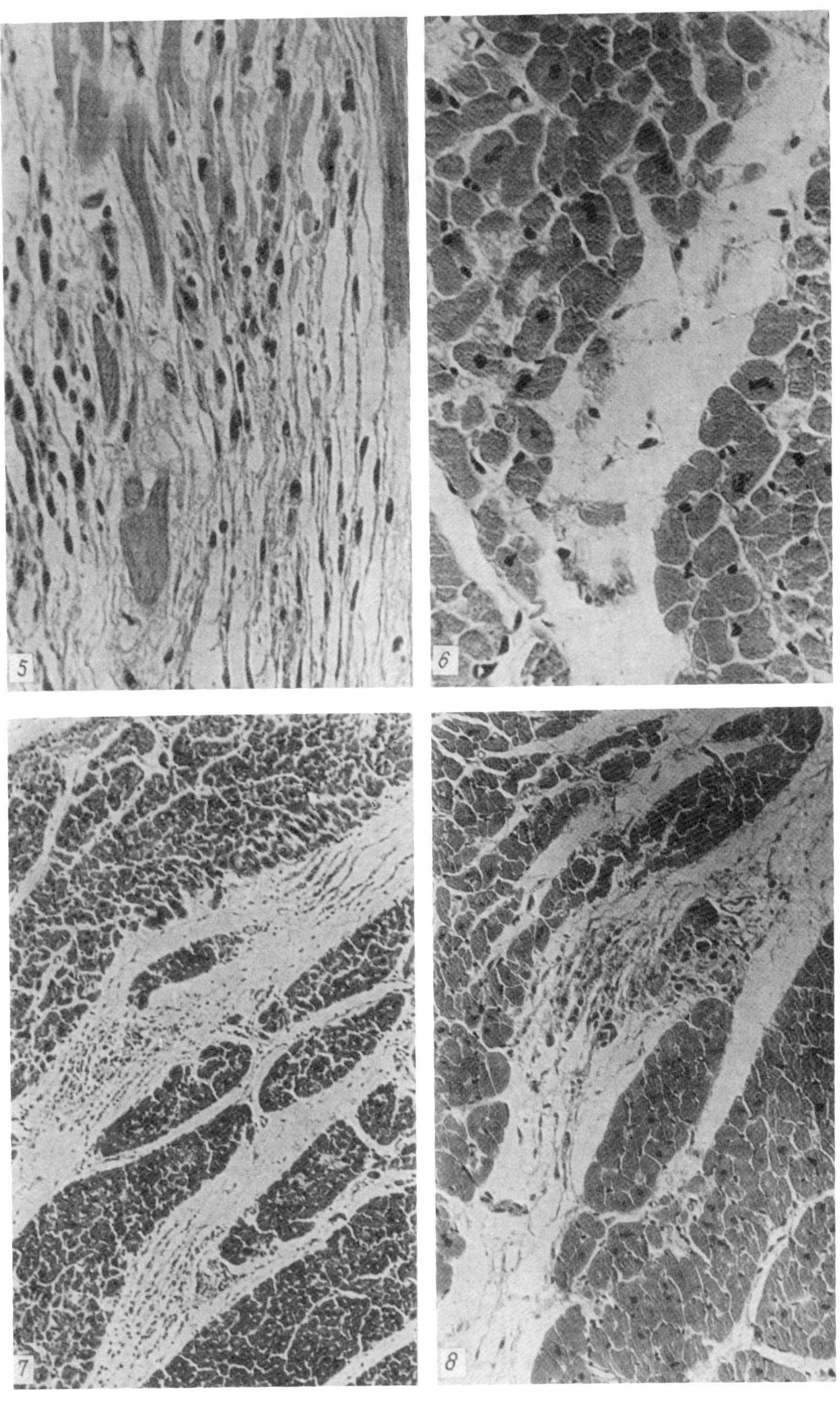

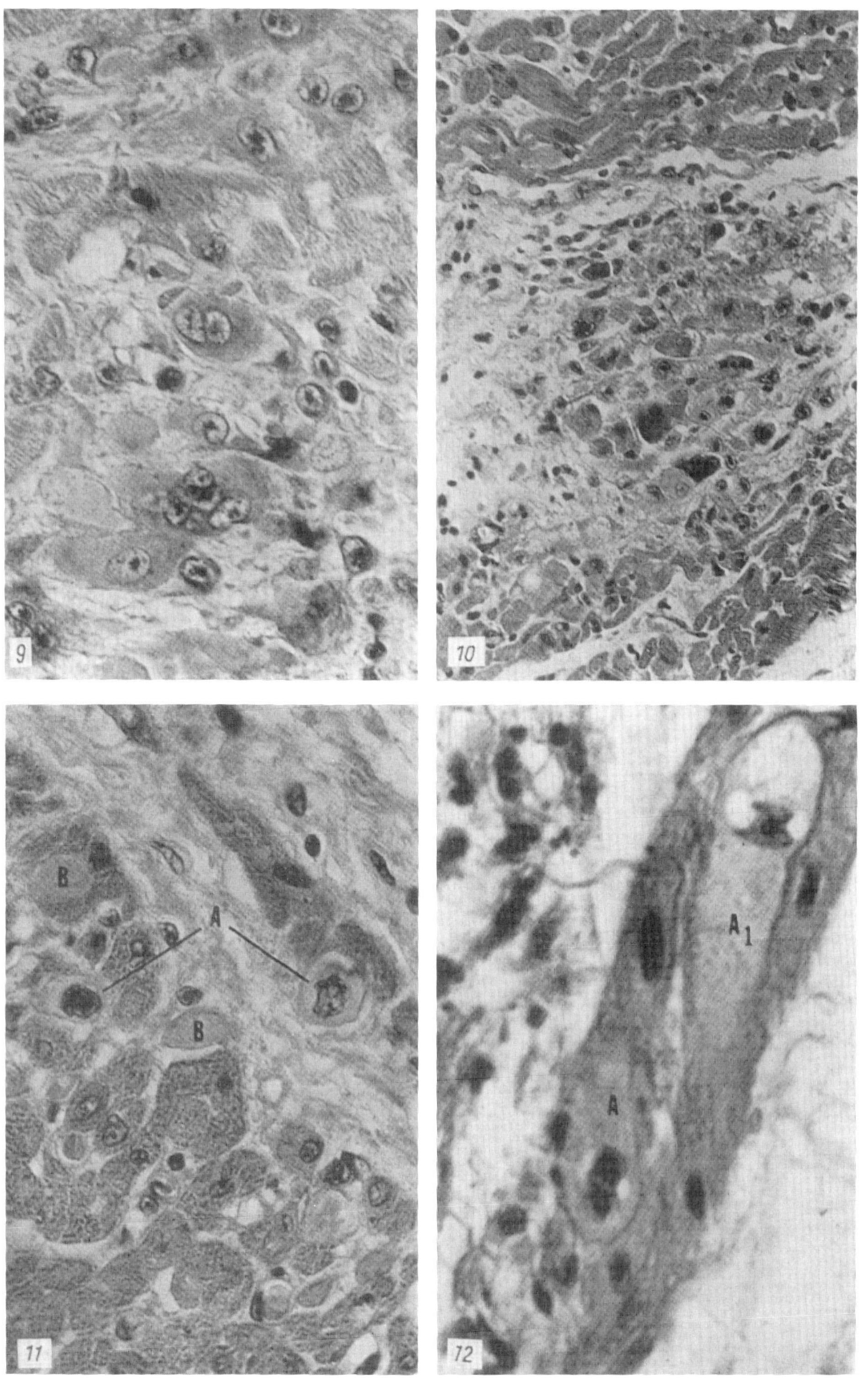
9
10
B
A
B
11
A₁
A
12

Type A cytogenesis of Aschoff cells through the stage of Anitschkow myocytes

This type of cytogenic process takes part in the formation of Anitschkow myocytes and subsequently owl eyed Aschoff cells (McDonald 1963). In the origin of Anitschkow myocytes (fig. 1), there may be seen a variety of degenerative changes such as fibrillary, fibrinoid, vacuolar or hydropic, and hyaline degeneration. Concomitant with degenerative changes in the myoplasm, the nuclei change their forms into those of Anitschkow myocytes which have been described in the literature as having a narrow, central chromatin bar with a serrated margin and clear nucleoplasm. In transverse section, these nuclei appear as a dark, central chromatin dot surrounded by clear nucleoplasm as shown in fig. 3 (C and D). Multinucleated owl eyed Aschoff cells, Type A, showing the nuclear characteristics of Anitschkow myocytes can be seen in fig. 4, where degenerated muscle element gives the appearance of fibrinoid. Our views on the formation and development of Anitschkow myocytes are in full agreement with Anitschkow's observations as shown in fig. 2 (ANITSCHKOW 1913) and also with those of VON ALBERTINI (1953), MURPHY and BECKER (1966), and SERCK-HANSSEN (1966). Often there is a strong suggestion of proliferation of Anitschkow myocytes by direct division or fragmentation of nuclei without division of the cytoplasm as shown in figs. 1 (F) and 3 (A). The authors agree with ANITSCHKOW (1913) who described the prominent role of these myocytes in cicatrization of myocardium.

Type B cytogenic process of Aschoff cells through the stage of dedifferentiated cells of cardiac muscle origin

This type of cytogenic change starts with the lysis of myocardial fibers (figs. 4—6) frequently forming cleft-like spaces (fig. 6). Like many others, the senior author herself formerly regarded these spaces as artifacts or edematous changes before the phenomenon of cellular lysis became apparent on critical study (GHOSH 1957, McDonald 1975).

Concomitant with the process of lysis, tiny, hyperchromatic, round or spindle-shaped nuclei appear within the cardiac muscle fibers, while the original muscle nuclei have disappeared. These phenomena may be visualized by studying the sections of myocardium passing through longitudinal (fig. 5) and transverse (figs. 4 and 6) planes of muscle fibers. Dedifferentiated nuclei accumulate shaggy, fibrinoid irregular cytoplasm in further development toward Aschoff body formation (figs. 7 and 8). The shaggy cytoplasm of these developing cells may turn into myoplasm with cross striations (figs. 8) and have characteristic affinity for muscle stains (figs. 13 and 14). In the Aschoff body, the degenerating myoplasm as well as the regenerating myoplasm before the development of cross striations may look like damaged collagen or fibrinoid. (For detailed study of this type of cytogenic process, the reader is referred to McDonald 1975.)

Figs. 9—12. Necropsy no. 8337 (see fig. 3).

Fig. 9. An Aschoff body with a preponderance of Type C Aschoff cells having large hyalinized cytoplasm and single or multiple large vesicular nuclei, frequently hypochromatic. Damaged muscle fibers at the bottom of the picture have formed fibrinoid material within the Aschoff body. HE, ×600.

Fig. 10. The polymorphic nature of the Aschoff body is shown with many Type C Aschoff cells, and a few of Type A with single or multiple nuclei of Anitschkow myocyte type. Many tiny dedifferentiated nuclei among the damaged muscle elements are also present. HE, ×260.

Fig. 11. Within the cardiac muscle fibers, the appearance of Type C Aschoff cells (A) with hyaline cytoplasm and vesicular nuclei. (B) points out a hyalinized mass within the altered muscle fiber, with a rim of recognizably striated myoplasm. The nuclei are not visible in this transverse plane. HE, ×600.

Fig. 12. Hyalinized muscle fibers in longitudinal plane in the formation of Type C Aschoff cells (A and Al). Note the wavy, fibrillary changes at the left edge of the muscle cell (A$_1$) and compare with (G) in fig. 1 and 16. HE, ×700.

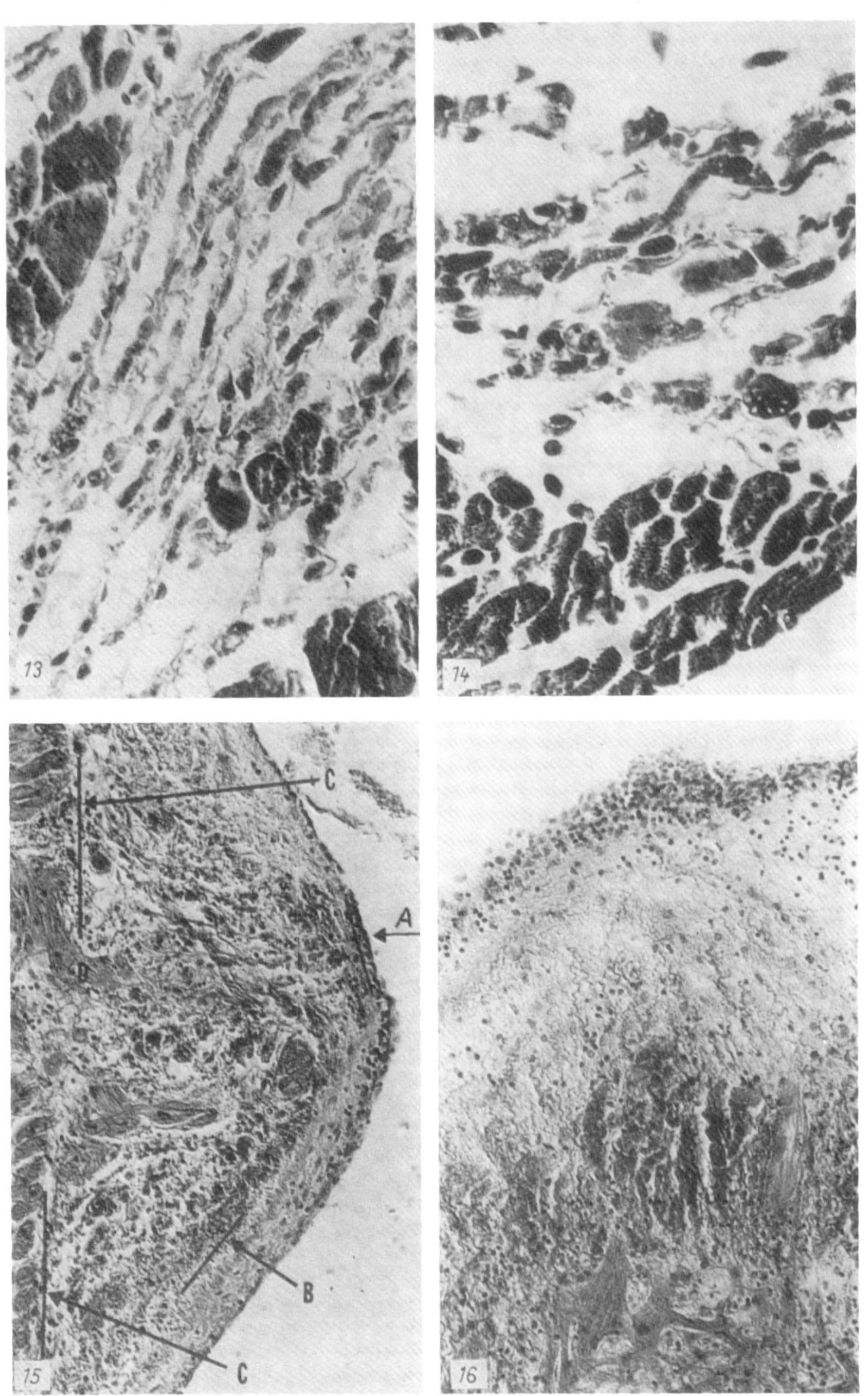

Type C cytogenesis of Aschoff cells from cardiac muscle fibers

In this category, mono- or multinucleated cells arise from damaged cardiac muscle fibers and usually have large vesicular nuclei and a light basophilic hyalinized cytoplasm when stained with hematoxylin and eosin. Good examples of this type Aschoff cell participating in Aschoff body formation are shown in figs. 9 and 10. The origin of this type of cell from cardiac muscle fibers associated with prominent hyaline degeneration can be appreciated by the study of figs. 11 and 12. Hyalinization of cardiac muscle fibers starts at the central part of the cells, while a rim of striated myoplasm may still be recognized at the periphery as shown in fig. 11 (B). Frequently the nucleus may be absent in transverse sections, because it occupies only a small part of the long, hyalinized muscle fibers (fig. 12).

It may be pointed out here that many cells derived from altered muscle fibers are usually designated as chronic inflammatory cells (figs. 5, 6, and 10). Cells formed from Anitschkow myocytes may appear similar to tissue neutrophils; this has been shown in a previous publication (McDONALD 1963).

It is apparent from this study that fibrinoid material, which is one of the components of Aschoff bodies, is a product of muscle degeneration (figs. 4, 5, 9, and 10) and that the regenerating myoplasm looks like fibrinoid material until it develops cross striations (figs. 8, 13, and 14). In addition to the regenerating muscle fibers in the Aschoff bodies, special stains also reveal collagenous fibers which may or may not be attached to the dedifferentiated nuclei or Anitschkow myocyte nuclei. These findings suggest the potential of myogenic cells to differentiate into fibrous connective tissue cells. This occurrence is at least partly responsible for the fibrous scarrings of myocardium in subacute and chronic cases. Occasionally one may find conspicuous fibrillary, fibrinoid, and hyaline degeneration of myocardium close to the endothelial lining where Aschoff bodies may or may not be found. On careful examination of fibrinoid material, one may find remainings of damaged muscle fibers (figs. 15 and 16) before they become completely unrecognizable and transformed into fibrous tissue. This may be the main process of formation of thickened endo- and subendocardium. Fibrous metaplasia is seen in other conditions of cardiac muscle (McDONALD 1962).

Figs. 13 and 14. Necropsy no. 5764 (see fig. 1). — Each of these photomicrographs illustrates regeneration or redifferentiation of cardiac muscle fibers with newly formed sarcoplasm inside the Aschoff body. Also noted is a small amount of tissue elements with the tinctorial characteristics of collagen, mostly connected with tiny, dedifferentiated nuclei and ill-defined Anitschkow myocyte nuclei.

Fig. 13. Verhoeff van Gieson stain. ×370.

Fig. 14. Masson's trichrome stain ×365.

Figs. 15 and 16. Necropsy no. 5283 (see fig. 5). The mechanism of formation of thickened endo- and subendocardium as a replacement of damaged cardiac muscle is shown in these figures. Fig. 15 demonstrates extensive fibrinoid and fibrillary degeneration of inner cardiac muscle between lines C and A; a few intact muscle fibers can be identified in the degenerating area. Line A is just beneath the endocardial lining cells. The beginning stages of thickened endocardium and thickened subendocardium formations can be seen in the upper right portion of the photomicrograph. In contrast, thickened endocardium has already formed to the right of line B. There is already a line of demarcation between myocardium and future subendocardium in the plane passing through lines C's. The demarcation plane is free of muscle fibers except for a small area (D). In fig. 16, wavy fibrillary material derived from degenerated muscle can be seen close to the inner border of the cardiac wall. Compare this fibrillary change with that of individual muscle fibers in fig. 1 (G) and fig. 12 (A).

Fig. 15. HE, ×140.

Fig. 16. HE, ×140.

Discussion

It is interesting to note that muscle fibers react in a variety of ways, and these reactions may result in the formation of cells of varied nature. Some of these cells may have the potential for further differentiation. This is shown in the case of dedifferentiated cells of myogenic origin and their potentials for muscle regeneration and collagenous fibrous tissue formation. We agree with ANITSCHKOW (1913) who described the prominent role of these myocytes (Anitschkow myocytes) in cicatrization of myocardium.

Some cells in myocardium which one would casually classify as inflammatory cells may have their origin in muscle fibers, as is evident in our figs. 5 and 6 and in earlier work (Mc DONALD 1963). It is a common experience of histologists, pathologists, and cytologists to frequently observe cells whose appearance does not conform to any of our cell classifications. Many of these may be cells in transition (GHOSH 1959, McDONALD 1962, 1968, 1970, 1975). SCHWANN (1847), who made a classical study of cells over a century ago, remarked, "Nature is very unwilling to accomodate herself to our schemes. The object of her aim is quite opposed to that of our intellect. She accords and accomodates all contrarites by gentle transition. The intellect disjoins and seeks everyhwere for strongly-marked contrasts."

As this paper presents, the changes in cardiac muscle in rheumatic fever involve a variety of degenerative processes. Subsequent to muscle degeneration, new types of cells evolve from damaged muscle fibers. Some of these cells fall into the category of Aschoff cells of Types A, B, and C derived by three different pathways from the same source material. The general belief that fibrinoid material of Aschoff bodies is of collagen origin may have been derived from the fact that the degenerating and regenerating eosinophilic muscle elements often give an appearance of damaged collagen (fibrinoid). We have observed that the degenerating muscle soon loses its affinity for muscle stains, and the regenerating muscle does not usually acquire the full affinity for these stains, almost until the cross striations are developed.

The preconceived idea that rheumatic fever is primarily a disease of collagen, has been partly responsible for the general neglect in viewing the actual changes in cardiac muscle fibers, even though in acute cases the clinical picture is more compatible with muscle damage than collagen disease. The fact that in chronic and subacute cases one often sees Aschoff bodies surrounded by fibrous collagenous tissue may also be partly responsible for the deduction of the theory that Aschoff bodies arise from collagenous tissues. The latter is the product of imperfect healing processes rather than the primary tissue for the origin of Aschoff bodies. ASCHOFF (1939) said in his last article, "It is in no way essential that the formation of the richly cellular nodules should be preceded by fibrinoid degeneration of ground substance." Mentioning a case of rheumatic fever which led to the death of a six year old boy, Aschoff confirmed that there was no trace of ground substance in Aschoff bodies. It may be mentioned here that there is very little collagenous tissue in the normal, healthy myocardium, especially in children.

Myogenic origin of Aschoff bodies and regeneration of cardiac muscle from Aschoff cells have been demonstrated with photomicrographys as early as 1920 by WHITMAN and EASTLAKE, and later by MURPHY (1952, 1959), GHOSH (1957), and McDONALD (1975). Within the Aschoff bodies, there appears to be an abortive attempt for muscle regeneration which is peculiar to rheumatic fever. The regeneration of cardiac muscle in general has been overlooked. This may be due to the fact that similar to skeletal muscle, mitosis rarely occurs in cardiac muscle. It has been shown in previous studies (McDONALD 1975) that dedifferentiated cells arising from lysing muscle fibers, with or without disruption of sacrcolemma, may redifferentiate into normal cardiac muscle fibers. These observations on regeneration of cardiac muscle agree with the parallel observations made by SPEIDEL (1938) in skeletal muscle. The tiny, hyperchromic dedifferentiated cells with potentials for regeneration may be called "cells in seed state". These cells, which may easily be confused with lymphocytes, may be analogous to the "satellite cells" of skeletal muscle with potential for regeneration as described by MAURO (1961), WALKER (1963) and CHURCH (1970).

194

Acknowledgements

The authors express grateful thanks to Dr. LAUREN V. ACKERMAN, formerly Professor of Surgical, Pathology, Washington University School of Medicine for his encouragement in this study, and to Dr. HENDLEY A. McDONALD for his assistance in the preparation of the manuscript.

The authors greatly appreciate the permission given by the Editors and the Publishers of the Journal of Clinical Pathology and the Journal of the Texas Medical Society for reproduction of the necessary photomicrographys.

Literature

ANITSCHKOW, N., Experimentelle Untersuchungen über die Neubildung des Granulationsgewebes im Herzmuskel. Beitr. path. Anat. allg. Pathol. **55**, 373–415 (1913).

ASCHOFF, L., The rheumatic nodules in the heart. Ann. Rheum. Dis. **1**, 161–166 (1939).

CHURCH, J. C. T., Cell population in skeletal muscle after regeneration. J. Embryol. Exp. Morph. **23**, 531—537 (1970).

GHOSH, HEMPROVA. See McDONALD, HEMPROVA GHOSH.

KRÖSING, R., Über die Rückbildung und Entwicklung der quergestreiften Muskelfasern. Virchows Arch. path. Anat. **128**, 445—484 (1892).

McDONALD, HEMPROVA GHOSH, Observations on the histogenesis of rheumatic lesions of the heart. (Abstract). Amer. J. Path. **33**, 598—599 (1957).

— Active cellular lysis, a phenomenon of growth process and its role in the formation of different epithelial patterns as shown in mammary carcinomas in mice. Brit. J. Cancer **13**, 200—207 (1959).

— Evidences in favor of fibrous metaplasia of cardiac muscle fibers in cases of gradual diminution of vascular supply. (Abstract). Anat. Rec. **142**, 318 (1962).

— Origin of Anitschkow's myocytes from cardiac muscle fibers. Texas State J. Med. **59**, 1062—1067 (1963).

— Origin of vascular channels from epithelial tissue as shown in livers. J. Am. Medical Women's Assoc. **23**, 545—553 (1968).

— Structural changes in malignant epithelial cells suggesting stroma formation as shown in mammary carcinomas in mice. J. Am. Medical Women's Assoc. (Woman Physician). **25**, 493—501 (1970).

— Myocardial lysis in acute rheumatic fever followed by regeneration of cardiac muscle and origin of Aschoff bodies. J. Clin. Path. **28**, 568—575 (1975).

MAURO, A., Satellite cells of skeletal muscle fibers. J. Biophys. Biochem. Cytol. **9**, 494—495 (1961).

MURPHY, G. E., Evidence that Aschoff bodies of rheumatic myocarditis develop from injured myofibers. J. Exptl. Med. **95**, 329—332 (1952).

— On muscle cells, Aschoff bodies, and cardiac failure in rheumatic heart disease. Bull. New York Acad. Med. **35**, 621—651 (1959).

— and C. G. BECKER, Occurrence of caterpillar nuclei within normal immature and normal appearing and altered mature heart muscle cells and the evolution of Anitschkow myocytes from the latter. Amer. J. Path. **48**, 931—958 (1966).

SCHWANN, T., Microscopical researches into the accordance in the structures and growth of animals and plants. Translated and published by Sydenham Society, London 1847.

SERCK-HANSSEN, A., The Anitschkow myocyte. Further evidence of its myogenic origin and non--rheumatic genesis. Acta Path. et Microbiol. Scandinav **66**, 471—477 (1966).

SPEIDEL, C. C., Studies of living muscles; I. Growth, injury and repair of striated muscle, as revealed by prolonged observations of individual fibers in living frog tadpoles. Amer. J. Anat. **62**, 179—235 (1938).

VON ALBERTINI, A., Zur Pathogenese des Rheumatischen Granuloms. Schweizer. Med. Wochenschr. **83**, 772—776 (1953).

WALKER, B. E., The origin of myoblasts and the problem of dedifferentiation. Exp. Cell Res. **30**, 80—92 (1963).

WHITMAN, R. C., and A. C. EASTLAKE, Rheumatic myocarditis. Arch. Int. Med. **26**, 601—611 (1920),